600 KETO DIET COOKBOOK

Delicious Low-carb Ketogenic Recipes for Beginners and Advanced Users to Lose Weight Fast

Danel Karol

Table of Content

Part I The Keto Diet Basics

A typical keto diet usually consists of foods high in healthy fats and protein, including red meat and poultry, non-starchy vegetables, fatty fish, dark, keto-style coffee, leafy greens, bone and broths just to name a few. For someone just starting on Keto, it can be challenging to follow a low carb diet.

Which Keto Diet Should Be Your Kind?

You know, you can't throw yourself in there and follow what stay-at-home mom dieters or "I tried it for only two weeks" dieters throw out there for you to follow. They might not be wrong, but it is better when you understand your goals, body type, and ideas concerning the diet. You might want to ask yourself these questions:

Are you dieting to feel clean, be healthy, and look attractive while using the keto diet as a tool for this goal?

Or maybe you desire a Tim McGraw/ Ellie Goulding fit kind of a body figure and would rather have that than just eat healthily?

Probably, you were spoiled with many types of meats growing up and just transitioning from the carnivore diet to keto seems sturdy. Will you instead transition slowly with more meats for your consumption?

Four scientific ways group the keto diet and trust me; they help you achieve any of the above goals by adjusting the diets slightly.

◇ The Standard Ketogenic Diet (SKD)

I'll term this type the butter and mixed seed bread of the keto diet, which combines the basic rules of the diet for anyone starting freshly. It is a combination of 75% and more healthy fats, 20% to 30% of proteins, and not exceeding 5% of carbohydrates in a daily meal. Meaning, in a day, your total net carb intake should not exceed 30 grams while your caloric intake may fluctuate based on the ingredients used in your meals.

This option will transition you smoothly into ketosis while keeping you healthy, shedding fat accurately, but will not be concerned with building muscles. I am an SKD kind of a keto dieter.

◇ The Targeted Ketogenic Diet (TKD)

If you frequent the gym often and work out more intensely than regular cardio exercises, then the TKD will be yours.

For the sake of having more energy for your workouts, you will have to stick to the SKD, but 30 minutes before your workout, you are open to consuming 25 to 30 grams of carbohydrates to increase your energy levels for all the weight lifting and intense jumps.

◇ The Cyclical Ketogenic Diet (CKD)

For bodybuilding, here's the way to go!

Your body will require a lot more protein to build muscles. Mind you, carbs do not build muscles, but protein.

Working with a ratio of six days of clean ketoing to one day of wild carb feasting every week, this type of keto lifestyle will fill your glycogen stores to support the building of muscles for the result that you seek.

Increase your protein intake by 5% to 10% once or twice a week to drive the muscle-building pace. Be sure to tally this choice with medical advice, so that you can remain in ketosis.

◇ The High Protein Ketogenic Diet (HPKD)

More sidelined to the carnivorous kind of keto dieting, I do not find many dieters interested in this form of diet; however, it is essential that you're aware. It is a choice for extreme meat lovers and bodybuilders, which exceeds the CKD by some excess protein intake. On this diet, your macros become 60% of healthy fats, 35% of protein, and 5% of carbohydrates. For effective ketosis results, this diet should be practiced interchangeably with the SKD to drive the consistent production of ketones by the liver.

Do you know, which fits you best yet?

The Benefits of The Keto Diet

Count me a liar if I hailed the keto diet so hard, making it look like that one magical opportunity that will make you live forever. While loaded with so many benefits, which makes it one of the best diets currently (that I am super excited to share), it sure has its side effects that are tremendously controllable and avoidable.

Let's explore the right sides first, and then we can move on to the others:

◇ Weight Loss Quickly

Shedding off the fat on the keto diet is as seamless and fast as it gets. When fats burn for fuel in the body, the realization is weight loss. In ketosis, your body switches from burning carbs for energy and uses stored fats to create energy. What happens? Insulin (the fat storing hormone) levels drop and release fats to get burning. Adversely, on a high carb diet, insulin levels increase, fats are stored in the body; hence, you begin to experience excessive weight gain.

◇ Mental Focus Improves

I know some co-dieters that love ketoing because of the mental focus that it offers. In ketosis, you focus better, concentrate more steadily, and use up your brain-racking abilities more effectively to solve problems. This improvement occurs because when ketones are a more consistent fuel provision to the brain, it is not yo-yoed while it works of which carbs will have caused.

◇ Energy Levels Increase Adequately

While still about fueling, fats are the most effective fuel-burning molecule that the body has. When burned into ketones, it sparks up the body with better, reliable, and steady energy that makes you do more in the same period than you will have done on a high-carb diet. Meanwhile, due to the satiety power of fats, your body feels full for extended periods, which aids in making you more energetic for your tasks.

◇ Your Crazy Cravings Are Curbed

Carbs are such deceit! They bug you with constant feelings of hunger because of their sugar content. No wonder on a high-carb diet when you feel hungry, you crave more carbs or sugars for satisfaction – I'll tell you that's the carbohydrate on a tricking spree. For this reason, I love the keto diet because fats keep you full for extended periods; hence, such crazy food desires to grab carb snacks is quickly curbed.

◇ Fights Type II Diabetes As Insulin Levels Decrease

By now, I am sure you are aware that excess sugars in the blood cause type II diabetes. Once insulin levels in the body fall from the increase of ketones, blood sugar automatically reduces, and then, HbA1c count lowers. This process stands the chance of healing diabetes, which in recent times has had miraculous testimonies of people with diabetes been recovered.

Side Effects of The Keto Diet

◇ Keto Flu

Keto flu is not a bad thing; so do not be alarmed when you experience this in the first week or two of keto dieting. You may experience feelings like headaches, weakness, nausea, confusion, irritability, and much more sometimes. These experiences are normal. Once the body begins burning fats into ketosis, it goes through a wear and repair process to adjust to the new way of eating and processing of nutrients. Hence, the flu-like symptoms that you feel. Meanwhile, during this period, you are likely to pass out urine frequently, which could lead to dehydration and sodium loss. It is crucial that you drink a lot of water mixed with a little salt to refill your water and sodium wells. You should also rest a lot more and avoid partaking in strenuous activities, especially on your weak days. This way, the body can recoup, use, and store energy more effectively.

◇ Possible Nutritional Deficiencies

Because the body focuses on high-carb foods, the possibility to lose out on some electrolytes and micronutrients is high. It is wise to seek a doctor's advice, run some tests, and support the diet with keto-safe foods and supplements that boost phytochemicals, minerals, fiber, calcium, etc. Also, mark out foods that give you allergies so that you do not double battle the keto flu and allergies in your early days of the keto diet.

◇ The Temptation to Fall back to Carbs

It is usually not a smooth ride in your first few days after you've fed on high carbs for most parts of your life. There is a high temptation rate to add a little extra rice to that plate of coconut shrimp curry instead of consuming cauliflower. Responding to such tricky demands by the body will only make you keto dirty and eventually draw you off the keto diet. To curb this desire, I like to advise a slow walk into the keto diet where you cut down on carbs gradually, day after day, and train the body to restrict carbs totally after a while. Starting with a reduction of about 5 grams per day is a good starting point to transition properly.

Also, design and stick to a keto meal plan, to prevent you from second-guessing your next meal, which could easily land you into the carb zone.

The Keto Eating Rules

"I really believe that the more informed you are about the benefits of a healthy bite versus the chain reaction that you're going to put into effect in your body when you take that bite—you just suddenly don't want to make that choice for yourself anymore. It's beyond willpower at that point; it's become a desire to do something good for yourself."

—Christie Brinkley

Eating on the keto diet requires a bit of planning, discipline, and adjustments. Since, you will no longer be feeding heavily on carbs, what then serves as replacements for the carb take-outs? Below I share a long list of things to exclude from the diet and then the foods to enjoy.

To achieve success will require a bit of planning around your eating patterns, food supply, budget, and schedules to ensure that your daily macro requirements are consistently on point.

◇ Foods Not to Eat

Start by cleaning your refrigerator and pantry of these foods because they are very high in carbs.

Tubers:

potatoes, sweet potatoes, yam, taro, etc.

Legumes & Grains:

Rice (in all forms), corn, millet, oats, barley, rye, lentils, soya beans, pasta, etc.

Flours:

all-purpose flour, self-rising flour, rice flour, etc.

Sugar-Concentrated Fruits:

Apples, banana, pawpaw, oranges, pineapple, mango, watermelon, kiwi, apricot, grapes, etc.

Sweet Treats:

Candies, additives, sweeteners, sweet drinks, etc.

◇ Foods to Eat

You will have to fill your kitchen with these items as your budget leads.

Green and above the Ground Vegetables:

Asparagus, spinach, kale, collards, zucchinis, rapini, mushrooms, bell peppers, cabbages, olives, onions, jalapenos, eggplants, tomatoes, green beans, cauliflower, Brussel sprouts, okra, arugula, bok choy, scallions, shallots, etc.

Some Root Vegetables:

These are less carb-concentrated but should be eaten in minimum quantities. Turnips, parsnips, pumpkin, radishes, butternut squash, kohlrabi, celeriac, etc.

High, healthy fats:

Olive oil, coconut oil, butter, ghee, tallow, avocados, fatty cheeses, heavy cream, sour cream, whipping cream, cooking cream, unsweetened almond milk, unsweetened coconut milk, unsweetened cashew milk, etc.

Seeds and Nuts:

Almonds, pistachios, pecans, cashew nuts, peanuts, sesame seeds, chia seeds, macadamia nuts, sunflower seeds, walnuts, pumpkin seeds, peanut butter, hemp seeds, etc.

Protein:

Red meats, poultry, seafood, soy chorizo, bacon, pancetta, tofu, tempeh, low-carb protein powders.

Herbs, Spices, and Seasonings:

Salt, black pepper, white pepper, parsley, thyme, tarragon, cloves, bay leaves, oregano, basil, rosemary, marjoram dill, chives, turmeric, coriander, garlic, ginger, red curry, cinnamon, pumpkin spice, cumin, etc.

Low-Carb Fruits:

Strawberries, blueberries, raspberries, blackberries, goji berries, coconut, and olives.

Safe Condiments:

Sugar-free versions of mayonnaise, Worcestershire sauce, barbecue sauce, maple syrup, tamarind sauce, mustard, salsa, marinara sauce, vinegar, lemon juice, chimichurri, homemade pesto, etc.

Drinks:

Water, tea, latte, coffee, lassi, berry smoothies, low-carb wines, fresh low carb fruit juices, etc.

◇ Replacement Ingredients:

The recipes contain some unfamiliar ingredients that may leave you guessing their identification. I clarify them in the categories below, which are also widely available in most big grocery stores for purchase.

Coconut and Almond Flour:

For all types of high-carb flours, these slightly flavored flours work magic. They are 100% low in carbs and for their flavor; they will usually make foods taste better than regular flour.

Swerve Sugar, Erythritol, and Low Carb Syrups:

These are naturally derived sugars with no calories, no carbs, are non-glycemic, non-GMO, and taste 80% like regular sugar, which replace all forms of regular sugars. You may find swerve sugar and sweeteners in white, brown, and confectionary versions.

Arrowroot Starch and Xanthan Gum:

Both options replace cornstarch as thickening agents for stews, soups, and drinks. They are very low in carbohydrates and do not alter the taste and flavor of foods.

Part II   Keto Recipes

Breakfast

Burrito

Prep Time: 10 minutes **Cook Time:** 16 minutes
Servings: 1

Ingredients:
1 teaspoon coconut oil
1 teaspoon garlic powder
1 teaspoon cumin
¼ pound ground beef
1 teaspoon sweet paprika
1 teaspoon onion powder
1 onion, peeled, and julienned
1 teaspoon fresh cilantro, chopped
Salt and ground black pepper, to taste
3 eggs

Directions:
1.Heat a pan over medium heat, add beef, and brown all over. Add salt, pepper, cumin, garlic, onion powder, and paprika, stir, cook for 4 minutes, and take off heat.
2.In a bowl, mix eggs with salt, pepper, and whisk. Heat a pan with oil over medium heat, add egg, spread evenly, and cook for 6 minutes.
3.Transfer the egg burrito to a plate, divide beef mixture, add onion and cilantro, roll, and serve.

Nutrition: Calories: 482, Fat: 24.8, Fiber: 2.4, Carbohydrates: 11.3, Protein: 52.2

Breakfast Hash

Prep Time: 10 minutes **Cook Time:** 16 minutes
Servings: 2

Ingredients:
1 tablespoon coconut oil
2 garlic cloves, peeled and minced
½ cup beef stock
Salt and ground black pepper, to taste
1 onion, peeled and chopped
2 cups corned beef, chopped
1 pound radishes, cut in quarters

Directions:
1.Heat up a pan with the oil over medium–high heat, add the onion, stir, and cook for 4 minutes.
2.Add radishes, stir, and cook for 5 minutes. Add garlic, stir, and cook for 1 minute.
3.Add stock, beef, salt, pepper, stir, cook for 5 minutes, take heat, and serve.

Nutrition: Calories: 316, Fat: 21.2, Fiber: 4.9, Carbohydrates: 13.9, Protein: 18

Brussels Sprout Delight

Prep Time: 10 minutes **Cook Time:** 12 minutes
Servings: 3

Ingredients:
3 eggs
Salt and ground black pepper, to taste
1 tablespoon butter, melted
2 shallots, peeled and minced
2 garlic cloves, peeled and minced
12 ounces Brussels sprouts, sliced thin
2 ounces bacon, chopped
1½ tablespoons apple cider vinegar

Directions:
1.Heat a pan over medium heat, add bacon, stir, cook until crispy, transfer to a plate and set aside.
2.Heat the pan again over medium heat, add shallots and garlic, stir, and cook for 30 seconds. Add Brussels sprouts, salt, pepper, apple cider vinegar, stir, and cook for 5 minutes.
3.Return bacon to pan, stir, and cook for 5 minutes. Add butter, stir, and make a hole in the center.
4.Crack eggs into pan, cook thoroughly, and serve.

Nutrition: Calories: 275, Fat: 16.5, Fiber: 4.3, Carbohydrates: 17.2, Protein: 17.4

Cereal Nibs

Prep Time: 10 minutes **Cook Time:** 45minutes
Servings: 4

Ingredients:
4 tablespoons hemp hearts
½ cup chia seeds
1 cup water
1 tablespoon vanilla extract
1 tablespoon psyllium powder
2 tablespoons coconut oil
1 tablespoon swerve
2 tablespoons cocoa nibs

Directions:
1.In a bowl, mix chia seeds with water, stir, and set aside for 5 minutes.
2.Add hemp hearts, vanilla extract, psyllium powder, oil, swerve and stir well with a mixer.
3.Add cocoa nibs and stir until you obtain a dough. Divide dough into 2 pieces, shape into cylinder form, place on a lined baking sheet, flatten well, cover with a parchment paper, place in an oven at 285ºF and bake for 20 minutes.
4.Remove parchment paper and bake for 25 minutes. Take cylinders out of oven, set aside to cool down, and cut into small pieces before serving.

Nutrition: Calories: 324, Fat: 25.4, Fiber: 8.1, Carbohydrates: 14.3, Protein: 12.8

Chia Pudding

Prep Time: 10 minutes **Cook Time:** 30 minutes
Servings: 2

Ingredients:
2 tablespoons coffee
2 cups water
⅓ cup chia seeds
1 tablespoon swerve
1 tablespoon vanilla extract
2 tablespoons cocoa nibs
⅓ cup coconut cream

Directions:
1.Heat a small pot with water over medium heat, bring to a boil, add coffee, simmer for 15 minutes, take off the heat and strain into a bowl.
2.Add vanilla extract, coconut cream, swerve, cocoa nibs, and chia seeds, stir well, keep in the refrigerator for 30 minutes, divide into 2 breakfast bowls and serve.

Nutrition: Calories: 149, Fat: 12.5, Fiber: 2.9, Carbohydrates: 10.8, Protein: 2

Hemp Porridge

Prep Time: 3 minutes **Cook Time:** 3 minutes
Servings: 1

Ingredients:
1 tablespoon chia seeds
1 cup almond milk
2 tablespoons flaxseeds
½ cup hemp hearts
½ teaspoon ground cinnamon
1 tablespoon stevia
¾ teaspoon vanilla extract
¼ cup almond flour
1 tablespoon hemp hearts, for serving

Directions:
1.In a pan, mix almond milk with ½ cup hemp hearts, chia seeds, stevia, flaxseeds, cinnamon, and vanilla extract, stir well, and heat over medium heat.
2.Cook for 2 minutes, take off heat, add almond flour, stir well, and pour into a bowl.
3.Top with 1 tablespoon hemp hearts, and serve.

Nutrition: Calories: 1030, Fat: 91.6, Fiber: 18.5, Carbohydrates: 32.7, Protein: 29.5

Simple Breakfast Cereal

Prep Time: 10 minutes **Cook Time:** 3 minutes
Servings: 2

Ingredients:
½ cup coconut, shredded
4 teaspoons butter
2 cups almond milk
1 tablespoon stevia
A pinch of salt
⅓ cup macadamia nuts, chopped
⅓ cup walnuts, chopped
⅓ cup flaxseed

Directions:
1.Heat a pot with butter over medium heat, add milk, coconut, salt, macadamia nuts, walnuts, flaxseed, stevia, and stir well.
2.Cook for 3 minutes, stir again, take off heat, and set aside for 10 minutes. Divide into 2 bowls, and serve.

Nutrition: Calories: 1078, Fat: 106.6, Fiber: 15.5, Carbohydrates: 26.8, Protein: 16.5

Simple Egg Porridge

Prep Time: 10 minutes **Cook Time:** 4 minutes
Servings: 2

Ingredients:
2 eggs
1 tablespoon stevia
⅓ cup heavy cream
2 tablespoons butter, melted
A pinch of ground cinnamon

Directions:
1.In a bowl, mix eggs with stevia and heavy cream, and whisk.
2.Heat a pan with butter over medium–high heat, add egg mixture, and cook until done.
3.Transfer to 2 bowls, sprinkle cinnamon on top, and serve.

Nutrition: Calories: 234, Fat: 23.3, Fiber: 0, Carbohydrates: 0.9, Protein: 6.1

Pancakes

Prep Time: 3 minutes **Cook Time:** 12 minutes
Servings: 4

Ingredients:
½ teaspoon ground cinnamon
1 teaspoon stevia
2 eggs
Vegetable oil cooking spray
2 ounces cream cheese

Directions:
1.In a blender, mix eggs with cream cheese, stevia, and cinnamon, and blend well.
2.Heat a pan with some cooking spray over medium–high heat, pour ¼ of the batter, spread well, cook for 2 minutes, flip, and cook for 1 minute.
3.Transfer to a plate, and repeat with the rest of the batter. Serve warm.

Nutrition: Calories: 82, Fat: 7.1, Fiber: 0.2, Carbohydrates: 1.3, Protein: 3.9

Breakfast in a Glass

Prep Time: 3 minutes **Cook Time:** 0 minutes
Servings: 2

Ingredients:
1 cup greens
¼ cup cocoa nibs
1 cup water
1 cup blueberries, frozen
¼ cup unsweetened cocoa powder
1 small avocado, pitted and peeled
¼ teaspoon turmeric

Directions:
1.In a blender, mix avocado with cocoa powder, blueberries, turmeric and blend well.
2.Add water, greens, and cocoa nibs, blend for 2 minutes, pour into glasses, and serve.

Nutrition: Calories: 299, Fat: 23.3, Fiber: 13.4, Carbohydrates: 27.9, Protein: 5.4

Almond Pancakes

Prep Time: 10 minutes **Cook Time:** 10 minutes
Servings: 12

Ingredients:
6 eggs
A pinch of salt
½ cup coconut flour
¼ cup stevia
⅓ cup coconut, shredded
½ teaspoon baking powder
1 cup almond milk
¼ cup coconut oil
1 teaspoon almond extract
¼ cup almonds, toasted
2 ounces cocoa powder
Vegetable oil cooking spray

Directions:
1.In a bowl, mix coconut flour with stevia, salt, baking powder, coconut, and stir. Add coconut oil, eggs, almond milk, almond extract, and stir well.
2.Add cocoa powder, almonds, and whisk again.
3.Heat a pan with cooking spray over medium heat, add 2 tablespoons batter, spread into a circle, cook until it's golden, flip, cook again until done, and transfer to a plate in a warm oven.
4.Repeat with the rest of the batter and serve right away.

Nutrition: Calories: 178, Fat: 14.6, Fiber: 5.3, Carbohydrates: 9.8, Protein: 5.6

Pumpkin Pancakes

Prep Time: 10 minutes **Cook Time:** 15 minutes
Servings: 6

Ingredients:
1 ounce egg white protein
2 ounces hazelnut flour
2 ounces flaxseeds, ground
1 teaspoon baking powder
1 cup coconut cream
1 tablespoon chai masala
1 teaspoon vanilla extract
½ cup pumpkin puree
3 eggs
5 drops stevia
1 tablespoon swerve
1 teaspoon coconut oil

Directions:
1.In a bowl, mix the flaxseeds with hazelnut flour, egg white protein, baking powder, chai masala, and stir.
2.In another bowl, mix coconut cream with vanilla extract, pumpkin puree, eggs, stevia, swerve, and stir.
3.Combine the 2 mixtures and stir well.
4.Heat a pan with oil over medium–high heat, pour 1/6 of the batter, spread into a circle, cover, reduce heat to low, cook for 3 minutes on each side, and transfer to a plate.
5.Keep warm, repeat with the rest of the batter, and serve right away.

Nutrition: Calories: 215, Fat: 16.9, Fiber: 4.3, Carbohydrates: 8.4, Protein: 8.7

Nutty Breakfast Smoothie

Prep Time: 5 minutes **Cook Time:** 0 minutes
Servings: 1

Ingredients:
2 brazil nuts
1 cup coconut milk
10 almonds
2 cups spinach leaves
1 teaspoon greens powder
1 teaspoon whey protein
1 tablespoon psyllium seeds
1 tablespoon potato starch

Directions:
1.In a blender, mix spinach with Brazil nuts, coconut milk, almonds and blend well.
2.Add green powder, whey protein, potato starch, psyllium seeds, and blend well.
3.Pour into a tall glass and serve.

Nutrition: Calories: 1096, Fat: 104.1, Fiber: 12.6, Carbohydrates: 35.5, Protein: 24

Waffles

Prep Time: 10 minutes **Cook Time:** 20 minutes
Servings: 5

Ingredients:
5 eggs, separated
3 tablespoons almond milk
1 teaspoon baking powder
3 tablespoons stevia
4 tablespoons coconut flour
2 teaspoon vanilla extract
4 ounces butter, melted

Directions:
1.In a bowl, whisk egg whites using a mixer. In another bowl, mix flour with stevia, baking powder, and egg yolks, and whisk.
2.Add vanilla extract, butter, milk, and stir well. Add egg whites and stir.
3.Pour some of the mixture into a waffle maker, and cook until golden. Repeat with the rest of the batter and serve the waffles right away.

Nutrition: Calories: 255, Fat: 25, Fiber: 0.5, Carbohydrates: 1.5, Protein: 6.1

Simple French Toast

Prep Time: 5 minutes **Cook Time:** 45 minutes
Servings: 18

Ingredients:
1 cup whey protein
12 egg whites
4 ounces cream cheese
For the French toast:
1 teaspoon vanilla extract
½ cup coconut milk
2 eggs
1 teaspoon ground cinnamon
½ cup butter, melted
½ cup almond milk
½ cup swerve

Directions:
1.In a bowl, mix 12 egg whites with a mixer for a few minutes.
2.Add protein and stir gently. Add cream cheese and stir again.
3.Pour into 2 greased bread pans, place in an oven at 325ºF, and bake for 45 minutes. Let bread to cool down, and slice into 18 pieces.
4.In a bowl, mix2 eggs with vanilla extract, cinnamon, and coconut milk, and whisk. Dip bread slices in this mixture.
5.Heat a pan with some coconut oil over medium heat, add bread slices, cook until golden on each side, and divide on plates.
6.Heat a pan with butter over high heat, add almond milk, and heat through. Add swerve, stir, and take off heat.
7.Leave aside to cool, and drizzle over French toast slices.

Nutrition: Calories: 124, Fat: 11.1, Fiber: 0.3, Carbohydrates: 5.3, Protein: 1.2

Baked Granola

Prep Time: 10 minutes **Cook Time:** 60 minutes
Servings: 4

Ingredients:
½ cup almonds, chopped
1 cup pecans, chopped
½ cup walnuts, chopped
½ cup coconut, flaked
¼ cup flax meal
½ cup almond milk
¼ cup sunflower seeds
½ cup stevia
¼ cup butter, melted
1 teaspoon vanilla extract
1 teaspoon ground cinnamon
½ teaspoon ground nutmeg
¼ cup water

Directions:
1.In a bowl, mix almonds with pecans, walnuts, coconut, flax meal, milk, sunflower seeds, butter, stevia, vanilla extract, cinnamon, salt, nutmeg, and water, and whisk.
2.Grease a baking sheet with parchment paper, spread granola mixture, and press well.
3.Cover with another piece of parchment paper, place in oven at 250ºF, and bake for 1 hour.
4.Take granola out of oven, set aside to cool down, break into pieces, and serve.

Nutrition: Calories: 516, Fat: 51.1, Fiber: 7.9, Carbohydrates: 11.9, Protein: 11

Kiwi and Strawberry Smoothie

Prep Time: 5 minutes **Cook Time:** 0 minutes
Servings: 6

Ingredients:
1 cup lettuce leaves
4 cups water
2 tablespoons fresh parsley
1 tablespoon fresh ginger, grated
1 tablespoon swerve
1 cup cucumber, sliced
½ avocado, pitted and peeled
½ cup kiwi, peeled and sliced
⅓ cup strawberries, chopped

Directions:
1.In a blender, mix the water with lettuce leaves, strawberries, parsley, cucumber, ginger, kiwi, avocado, and swerve, and blend well.
2.Pour into glasses and serve.

Nutrition: Calories: 53, Fat: 3.5, Fiber: 2, Carbohydrates: 5.8, Protein: 0.8

Steak and Eggs

Prep Time: 10 minutes **Cook Time:** 10 minutes
Servings: 1

Ingredients:
4 ounces sirloin steak
1 small avocado, pitted, peeled, and sliced
3 eggs
1 tablespoon butter
Salt and ground black pepper, to taste

Directions:
1.Heat a pan with butter over medium–high heat, crack eggs into pan, and cook them as you wish. Season with salt and pepper, take off heat, and transfer to a plate.
2.Heat another pan over medium–high heat, add steak, cook for 4 minutes, take off heat, set aside to cool down, and cut into thin strips.
3.Season with some salt and pepper and place next to the eggs. Add the avocado slices on the side and serve.

Nutrition: Calories: 911, Fat: 70.9, Fiber: 13.5, Carbohydrates: 18.3, Protein: 55

Chicken Quiche

Prep Time: 10 minutes **Cook Time:** 45 minutes
Servings: 5

Ingredients:
7 eggs
2 cups almond flour
2 tablespoons coconut oil
Salt and ground black pepper, to taste
2 zucchini, grated
½ cup heavy cream
1 teaspoon fennel seeds
1 teaspoon dried oregano
1 pound ground chicken

Directions:
1.In a food processor, blend almond flour with a pinch of salt. Add 1 egg, coconut oil and blend well.
2.Place dough in a greased pie pan and press well on the bottom.
3.Heat a pan over medium heat, add chicken, brown for a couple of minutes, take off heat, and leave aside.
4.In a bowl, mix 6 eggs with salt, pepper, oregano, cream, fennel seeds, and whisk. Add chicken and stir again.
5.Pour this into pie base, spread, place in an oven at 350ºF, and bake for 40 minutes. Let the pie to cool before slicing and serving.

Nutrition: Calories: 428, Fat: 28.6, Fiber: 2.4, Carbohydrates: 6.2, Protein: 27.7

Simple Smoothie Bowl

Prep Time: 5 minutes **Cook Time:** 0 minutes
Servings: 1

Ingredients:
2 ice cubes
1 tablespoon coconut oil
2 tablespoons heavy cream
1 cup spinach
½ cup almond milk
1 teaspoon protein powder
4 raspberries
1 tablespoon coconut, shredded
4 walnuts
1 teaspoon chia seeds

Directions:
1.In a blender, mix milk with spinach, cream, ice, protein powder, coconut oil, blend well, transfer to a bowl.
2.Top the bowl with raspberries, coconut, walnuts, chia seeds and serve.

Nutrition: Calories: 709, Fat: 66.9, Fiber: 11.7, Carbohydrates: 23.1, Protein: 14.4

Feta Omelet

Prep Time: 10 minutes **Cook Time:** 10 minutes
Servings: 1

Ingredients:
3 eggs
1 tablespoon butter
1 ounce feta cheese, crumbled
1 tablespoon heavy cream
1 tablespoon jarred pesto
Salt and ground black pepper, to taste

Directions:
1.In a bowl, mix eggs with heavy cream, salt, pepper, and whisk.
2.Heat a pan with butter over medium–high heat, add whisked eggs, spread into the pan, and cook the omelet until it's fluffy.
3.Sprinkle cheese and spread pesto on the omelet, fold in half, cover pan, and cook for 5 minutes. Transfer omelet to a plate and serve.

Nutrition: Calories: 474, Fat: 41.9, Fiber: 0, Carbohydrates: 3.1, Protein: 22.1

Breakfast Tuna Salad

Prep Time: 10 minutes **Cook Time:** 0 minutes
Servings: 4

Ingredients:
2 tablespoons sour cream
12 ounces canned tuna in olive oil
4 leeks, diced
Salt and ground black pepper, to taste
A pinch of red chili flakes
1 tablespoon capers
8 tablespoons mayonnaise

Directions:
1.In a salad bowl, mix tuna with capers, salt, pepper, leeks, chili flakes, sour cream, and mayonnaise.
2.Stir well and serve.

Nutrition: Calories: 377, Fat: 20.4, Fiber: 17., Carbohydrates: 20, Protein: 30.3

Chicken Omelet

Prep Time: 10 minutes **Cook Time:** 10 minutes
Servings: 1

Ingredients:
1 ounce rotisserie chicken, shredded
1 teaspoon mustard
1 tablespoon mayonnaise
1 tomato, cored and chopped
2 bacon slices, cooked and crumbled
2 eggs
1 small avocado, pitted, peeled, and chopped
Salt and ground black pepper, to taste

Directions:
1.In a bowl, mix the eggs with some salt and pepper and whisk.
2.Heat a pan over medium heat, spray with some cooking oil, add eggs, and cook omelet for 5 minutes.
3.Add chicken, avocado, tomato, bacon, mayonnaise, and mustard on one half of the omelet.
4.Fold the omelet, cover pan, and cook for 5 minutes. Transfer to a plate and serve.

Nutrition: Calories: 841, Fat: 69.1, Fiber: 14.2, Carbohydrates: 25, Protein: 26.5

Breakfast Meatloaf

Prep Time: 10 minutes **Cook Time:** 35 minutes
Servings: 4

Ingredients:
1 teaspoon butter
1 onion, peeled and chopped
1 pound sweet sausage, chopped
6 eggs
1 cup cheddar cheese, shredded
4 ounces cream cheese, softened
Salt and ground black pepper, to taste
2 tablespoons scallions, chopped

Directions:
1.In a bowl, mix eggs with salt, pepper, onion, sausage, half of the cream, and whisk.
2.Grease a loaf pan with butter, pour sausage and eggs mixture, place in an oven at 350ºF, and bake for 30 minutes.
3.Take meatloaf out of the oven, set aside for a couple of minutes, spread the rest of the cream cheese on top, and sprinkle the scallions and cheddar cheese all over.
4.Place meatloaf in oven again and bake for 5 minutes.
5.Then, place meatloaf under a broiler for 3 minutes, let it cool, slice it and serve.

Nutrition: Calories: 748, Fat: 62.8, Fiber: 0.7, Carbohydrates: 5.9, Protein: 38.8

Poached Eggs

Prep Time: 10 minutes **Cook Time:** 35 minutes
Servings: 4

Ingredients:
3 garlic cloves, peeled and minced
1 tablespoon butter
1 white onion, peeled and chopped
1 Serrano pepper, chopped
Salt and ground black pepper, to taste
1 red bell pepper, seeded and chopped
3 tomatoes, cored and chopped
1 teaspoon paprika
1 teaspoon cumin
¼ teaspoon chili powder
1 tablespoon fresh cilantro, chopped
6 eggs

Directions:
1.Heat a pan with butter over medium heat, add onion, stir, and cook for 10 minutes.
2.Add Serrano pepper and garlic, stir, cook for 1 minute. Add red bell pepper, stir, and cook for 10 minutes.
3.Add tomatoes, salt, pepper, chili powder, cumin, and paprika, stir, and cook for 10 minutes.
4.Crack eggs intopan, season with salt, and pepper, cover pan, and cook for 6 minutes.
5.Sprinkle cilantro and serve.

Nutrition: Calories: 180, Fat: 10,9, Fiber: 2,5, Carbohydrates: 10,5, Protein: 11,7

Breakfast Bowl

Prep Time: 10 minutes **Cook Time:** 20 minutes
Servings: 1

Ingredients:
4 ounces ground beef
1 onion, peeled and chopped
8 mushrooms, sliced
Salt and ground black pepper, to taste
2 eggs, whisked
1 tablespoon coconut oil
½ teaspoon smoked paprika
1 avocado, pitted, peeled, and chopped
12 black olives, pitted and sliced

Directions:
1.Heat a pan with coconut oil over medium heat, add onions, mushrooms, salt, and pepper, stir, and cook for 5 minutes.
2.Add beef, and paprika, stir, cook for 10 minutes, transfer to a bowl. Heat up the pan again over medium heat, add eggs, some salt, pepper, and scramble.
3.Return beef mixture to pan and stir. Add avocado and olives, stir, and cook for 1 minute. Transfer to a bowl and serve.

Nutrition: Calories: 1002, Fat: 74,9, Fiber: 19,4, Carbohydrates: 36,9, Protein: 55,6

Eggs and Sausages

Prep Time: 10 minutes **Cook Time:** 35 minutes
Servings: 6

Ingredients:
5 tablespoons butter
12 eggs
Salt and ground black pepper, to taste
1 ounce spinach, torn
12 ham slices
2 sausages, chopped
1 onion, peeled and chopped
1 red bell pepper, seeded and chopped

Directions:
1.Heat a pan with 1 tablespoon butter over medium heat, add sausages, onion, stir, and cook for 5 minutes.
2.Add bell pepper, salt, pepper, stir, and cook for 3 minutes, transfer to a bowl. Melt rest of the butter, and divide into 12 cupcake molds.
3.Add a slice of ham to each cupcake mold, divide spinach in each and then add sausage mixture.
4.Crack an egg on top, place in an oven, and bake at 425 degrees Fahrenheit for 20 minutes. Let them cool briefly before serving.

Nutrition: Calories: 378, Fat: 28,4, Fiber: 1,5, Carbohydrates: 6,2, Protein: 24,5

Frittata

Prep Time: 10 minutes **Cook Time:** 1 hour
Servings: 4

Ingredients:
9 ounces spinach
12 eggs
1 ounce pepperoni
1 teaspoon garlic, minced
Salt and ground black pepper, to taste
5 ounces mozzarella cheese, shredded
½ cup Parmesan cheese, grated
½ cup ricotta cheese
4 tablespoons olive oil
A pinch of nutmeg

Directions:
1.Squeeze liquid from spinach and put spinach in a bowl. In another bowl, mix eggs with salt, pepper, nutmeg, garlic, and whisk.
2.Add spinach, Parmesan cheese, ricotta cheese, and whisk.
3.Pour mixture into a pan, sprinkle with mozzarella cheese and pepperoni on top, place in oven, and bake at 375ºF for 45 minutes.
4.Let frittata cool down for a few minutes before serving.

Nutrition: Calories: 525, Fat: 40,7, Fiber: 1,4, Carbohydrates: 6,7, Protein: 35,9

Smoked Salmon Breakfast

Prep Time: 10 minutes **Cook Time:** 10 minutes
Servings: 3

Ingredients:
4 eggs, whisked
½ teaspoon avocado oil
4 ounces smoked salmon, chopped
For the sauce:
1 cup coconut milk
½ cup cashews, soaked and drained
¼ cup green onions, chopped
1 teaspoon garlic powder
Salt and ground black pepper, to taste
1 tablespoon lemon juice

Directions:
1.In a blender, mix cashews with coconut milk, garlic powder, lemon juice and blend well.
2.Add salt, pepper, and green onions, blend again, transfer to a bowl, and place in refrigerator.
3.Heat up a pan with oil over medium–low heat, add eggs, whisk, and cook until they are almost done. Place under a preheated broiler, and cook until eggs are set.
4.Divide the eggs on plates, top with smoked salmon, and serve with the green onion sauce on top.

Nutrition: Calories: 448, Fat: 37,3, Fiber: 2,7, Carbohydrates: 13,1, Protein: 19,8

Feta and Asparagus Delight

Prep Time: 10 minutes **Cook Time:** 25 minutes
Servings: 2

Ingredients:
12 asparagus spears
1 tablespoon olive oil
2 green onions, chopped
1 garlic clove, peeled and minced
6 eggs
Salt and ground black pepper, to taste
½ cup feta cheese

Directions:
1.Heat a pan with some water over medium heat, add asparagus, cook for 8 minutes, drain well, chop 2 spears, and reserve the rest.
2.Heat a pan with oil over medium heat, add garlic, chopped asparagus, onions, stir, and cook for 5 minutes. Add eggs, salt, pepper, stir, cover, and cook for 5 minutes.
3.Arrange asparagus spears on top of the frittata, sprinkle cheese, place in oven at 350ºF, and bake for 9 minutes. Divide on plates and serve.

Nutrition: Calories: 384, Fat: 28.3, Fiber: 3.4, Carbohydrates: 9.7, Protein: 25.5

Eggs Baked in Avocados

Prep Time: 10 minutes **Cook Time:** 20 minutes
Servings: 4

Ingredients:
2 avocados, cut in half and pitted
4 eggs
Salt and ground black pepper, to taste
1 tablespoon fresh chives, chopped

Directions:
1.Scoop some flesh from the avocado halves and arrange in a baking dish.
2.Crack an egg in each avocado, season with salt, pepper, place in oven at 425ºF, and bake for 20 minutes. Sprinkle chives at end and serve.

Nutrition: Calories: 268, Fat: 24, Fiber: 6.7, Carbohydrates: 9, Protein: 7.5

Breakfast Stir–fry

Prep Time: 10 minutes **Cook Time:** 30 minutes
Servings: 2

Ingredients:
½ pounds minced beef
2 teaspoons red chili flakes
1 tablespoon tamari sauce
2 bell peppers, seeded and chopped
1 teaspoon chili powder
1 tablespoon coconut oil
Salt and ground black pepper, to taste
For the bok choy:
6 bunches bok choy, trimmed and chopped
1 teaspoon fresh ginger, grated
Salt, to taste
1 tablespoon coconut oil
For the eggs:
1 tablespoon coconut oil
2 eggs

Directions:
1.Heat a pan with 1 tablespoon coconut oil over medium–high heat, add beef, bell peppers, stir, and cook for 10 minutes.
2.Add salt, pepper, tamari sauce, chili flakes, chili powder, stir, cook for 4 minutes, and take off heat.
3.Heat another pan with 1 tablespoon oil over medium heat, add bok choy, stir, and cook for 3 minutes.
4.Add salt, ginger, stir, cook for 2 minutes, and take off heat. Heat third pan with 1 tablespoon oil over medium heat, crack eggs into pan and fry them.
5.Divide beef and bell pepper mixture into 2 bowls. Divide bok choy and top with the eggs.

Nutrition: Calories: 510, Fat: 32.6, Fiber: 3.4, Carbohydrates: 13.1, Protein: 43.4

Scrambled Eggs

Prep Time: 10 minutes **Cook Time:** 10 minutes
Servings: 1

Ingredients:
4 bell mushrooms, chopped
3 eggs, whisked
Salt and ground black pepper, to taste
2 ham slices, chopped
¼ cup red bell pepper, seeded and chopped
½ cup spinach, chopped
1 tablespoon coconut oil

Directions:
1.Heat a pan with half of the oil over medium heat, add mushrooms, spinach, ham, bell pepper, stir, and cook for 4 minutes.
2.Heat another pan with the rest of the oil over medium heat, add eggs and scramble.
3.Add vegetables, ham, salt, and pepper, stir, cook for 1 minute, and serve.

Nutrition: Calories: 430, Fat: 31,9, Fiber: 2,4, Carbohydrates: 9, Protein: 29,5

Seasoned Hard Boiled Eggs

Prep Time: 10 minutes **Cook Time:** 4 minutes
Servings: 12

Ingredients:
4 tea bags
4 tablespoons salt
12 eggs
2 tablespoons ground cinnamon
6star anise
1 teaspoon ground black pepper
1 tablespoon peppercorns
8 cups water
1 cup tamari sauce

Directions:
1.Put water in a pot, add eggs, bring to a boil over medium heat, and cook until hard boiled.
2.Allow to cool and crack them without peeling. In a large pot, mix water with tea bags, salt, pepper, peppercorns, cinnamon, star anise, and tamari sauce.
3.Add cracked eggs, cover pot, bring to a simmer over low heat, and cook for 30 minutes. Discard tea bags and cook eggs for 3 hours and 30 minutes.
4.Let the eggs cool, peel, and serve.

Nutrition: Calories: 122, Fat: 4.6, Fiber: 0.8, Carbohydrates: 6.7, Protein: 13.9

Mexican Breakfast

Prep Time: 10 minutes **Cook Time:** 30 minutes
Servings: 8

Ingredients:
½ cup tomato paste
½ tsp garlic powder
1 tsp dried basil
1 tsp dried oregano
1 tsp cumin
2 tsp chili powder
1 pound ground pork
1 pound chorizo, chopped
Salt and ground black pepper, to taste
8 eggs
1 tomato, cored and chopped
3 tablespoons butter
½ cup onion, chopped
1 avocado, pitted, peeled, and chopped

Directions:
1.In a bowl, mix spices and tomato paste to make enchilada sauce. In a second bowl, mix pork with chorizo, stir, and spread on a lined baking sheet.
2.Spread enchilada sauce on top, place in oven at 350ºF, and bake for 20 minutes.
3.Heat a pan with butter over medium heat, add eggs, and scramble them.
4.Take pork mixture out of oven and spread scrambled eggs over them.
5.Sprinkle salt, pepper, tomato, onion, and avocado on top, divide on plates, and serve.

Nutrition: Calories: 513, Fat: 37.6, Fiber: 2.8, Carbohydrates: 8.4, Protein: 35.6

Shrimp and Bacon Breakfast

Prep Time: 10 minutes **Cook Time:** 15 minutes
Servings: 4

Ingredients:
1 cup mushrooms, sliced
4 bacon slices, chopped
4 ounces smoked salmon, chopped
4 ounces shrimp, deveined
Salt and ground black pepper, to taste
½ cup coconut cream

Directions:
1.Heat a pan over medium heat, add bacon, stir, and cook for 5 minutes.
2.Add mushrooms, stir, and cook for 5 minutes. Add salmon, stir, and cook for 3 minutes.
3.Add shrimp and cook for 2 minutes.
4.Add salt, pepper, and coconut cream, stir, cook for 1 minute, take off heat, and divide on plates.

Nutrition: Calories: 242, Fat: 16.8, Fiber: 0.8, Carbohydrates: 2.9, Protein: 19.9

Breakfast Pie

Prep Time: 10 minutes **Cook Time:** 45 minutes
Servings: 8

Ingredients:
½ onion, peeled and chopped
½ red bell pepper, seeded and chopped
¾ pound ground beef
Salt and ground black pepper, to taste
3 tablespoons taco seasoning
½ cup fresh cilantro, chopped
8 eggs
1 teaspoon coconut oil
For pie crust:
7 oz almond flour
2 oz coconut flour
1/2 tsp xanthan gum
1/2 tsp baking powder
6 oz butter (must be cold)
1 teaspoon baking soda

Directions:
1.Heat a pan with oil over medium heat, add beef, cook until it browns, and mix with salt, pepper, and taco seasoning.
2.Stir again, transfer to a bowl and set aside. Heat the pan again over medium heat with cooking juices from the meat, add onion and bell pepper, stir, and cook for 4 minutes. Add eggs, baking soda, and some salt, and stir well.
3.Add cilantro, stir again, and take off heat. In a large bowl mix pie crust ingredients. Store the mixture in the fridge for 1 hour.
4.Roll the pastry, place your baking dish on top of the pastry and flip them both up the right way.
5.Spread beef mixture in pie crust; add vegetables mixture, spread over meat, place in an oven at 350ºF, and bake for 45 minutes.
6.Let pie cool, slice, divide on plates, and serve with papaya slices.

Nutrition: Calories: 421, Fat: 34.8, Fiber: 2.7, Carbohydrates: 6.3, Protein: 23.3

Breakfast Skillet

Prep Time: 10 minutes **Cook Time:** 30 minutes
Servings: 4

Ingredients:
8 ounces mushrooms, chopped
Salt and ground black pepper, to taste
1 pound minced pork
1 tablespoon coconut oil
½ teaspoon garlic powder
½ teaspoon dried basil
2 tablespoons Dijon mustard
2 zucchini, chopped

Directions:
1.Heat a pan with oil over medium–high heat, add mushrooms, stir, and cook for 4 minutes.
2.Add zucchini, salt, pepper, stir, and cook for 4 minutes. Add pork, garlic powder, basil, pinch of salt and pepper, stir, and cook until meat is done.
3.Add mustard, stir, cook for 3 minutes, divide into bowls and serve.

Nutrition: Calories: 225, Fat: 8, Fiber: 1.9, Carbohydrates: 5.6, Protein: 33

Breakfast Casserole

Prep Time: 10 minutes **Cook Time:** 40 minutes
Servings: 4

Ingredients:
10 eggs
1 pound pork sausage, chopped
1 onion, peeled and chopped
3 cups spinach, torn
Salt and ground black pepper, to taste
3 tablespoons avocado oil

Directions:
1.Heat a pan with 1 tablespoon oil over medium heat, add sausage, stir, and brown it for 4 minutes.
2.Add onion, stir, and cook for 3 minutes. Add spinach, stir, and cook for 1 minute.
3.Grease a baking dish with the rest of the oil, and spread the sausage mixture in it.
4.Whisk eggs and add them to sausage mixture.
5.Stir gently, place in oven at 350ºF, and bake for 30 minutes. Let the casserole cool for a few minutes before serving.

Nutrition: Calories: 572, Fat: 44.5, Fiber: 1.6, Carbohydrates: 4.8, Protein: 36.9

Sausage Patties

Prep Time: 10 minutes **Cook Time:** 10 minutes
Servings: 4

Ingredients:
1 pound minced pork
Salt and ground black pepper, to taste
¼ teaspoon dried thyme
½ teaspoon dried sage
¼ teaspoon ground ginger
3 tablespoons cold water
1 tablespoon coconut oil

Directions:
1.Put meat in a bowl. In another bowl, mix water with salt, pepper, sage, thyme, and ginger, and whisk.
2.Add this to the meat, and stir well. Shape patties and place on a working surface.
3.Heat up a pan with coconut oil over medium–high heat, add patties, fry them for 5 minutes, flip, and cook them for 3 minutes. Serve warm.

Nutrition: Calories: 191, Fat: 7.4, Fiber: 0, Carbohydrates: 0, Protein: 29.7

Baked Eggs with Sausage

Prep Time: 10 minutes **Cook Time:** 40 minutes
Servings: 6

Ingredients:
1 pound sausage, chopped
1 leek, chopped
8 eggs, whisked
¼ cup coconut milk
6 asparagus stalks, chopped
1 tablespoon fresh dill, chopped
Salt and ground black pepper, to taste
¼ teaspoon garlic powder
1 tablespoon coconut oil, melted

Directions:
1.Heat a pan over medium heat, add sausage pieces, and brown for a few minutes.
2.Add asparagus and leek, stir, and cook for a few minutes. In a bowl, mix eggs with the salt, pepper, dill, garlic powder, coconut milk, and whisk.
3.Pour into a baking dish greased with coconut oil. Add sausage and vegetables on top and whisk.
4.Place in oven at 325ºF and bake for 40 minutes. Serve warm.

Nutrition: Calories: 397, Fat: 32, Fiber: 1, Carbohydrates: 4, Protein: 23.1

Sausage Quiche

Prep Time: 10 minutes **Cook Time:** 40 minutes
Servings: 6

Ingredients:
12 ounces pork sausage, chopped
Salt and ground black pepper, to taste
2 teaspoons whipping cream
2 tablespoons fresh parsley, chopped
10 mixed cherry tomatoes, halved
6 eggs
2 tablespoons Parmesan cheese, grated
5 eggplant slices

Directions:
1.Spread sausage pieces on a baking dish. Lay eggplant slices on top and add cherry tomatoes.
2.In a bowl, mix eggs with salt, pepper, cream, and Parmesan cheese, and whisk.
3.Pour into the baking dish, place in oven at 375ºF, bake for 40 minutes, and serve.

Nutrition: Calories: 275, Fat: 21.5, Fiber: 0.4, Carbohydrates: 1.9, Protein: 17.7

Chorizo and Cauliflower Breakfast

Prep Time: 10 minutes **Cook Time:** 45 minutes
Servings: 4

Ingredients:
1 pound chorizo, chopped
12 ounces canned green chilies, chopped
1 onion, peeled and chopped
½ teaspoon garlic powder
Salt and ground black pepper, to taste
1 cauliflower head, separated into florets
4 eggs, whisked
2 tablespoons green onions, chopped

Directions:
1.Heat a pan over medium heat, add chorizo, onion, stir, and brown for a few minutes.
2.Add green chilies, stir, cook for a few minutes, and take off heat. In a food processor, mix cauliflower with some salt and pepper and blend.
3.Transfer to a bowl, add eggs, salt, pepper, garlic powder, and chorizo mixture, whisk, transfer to a greased baking dish.
4.Bake in oven at 375ºF for 40 minutes. Let casserole cool down for a few minutes, sprinkle green onions on top, slice, and serve.

Nutrition: Calories: 883, Fat: 52.8, Fiber: 26.7, Carbohydrates: 68.2, Protein: 43.5

Italian Spaghetti Casserole

Prep Time: 10 minutes **Cook Time:** 55 minutes
Servings: 4

Ingredients:
4 tablespoons butter
1 spaghetti squash, halved
Salt and ground black pepper, to taste
½ cup tomatoes, cored and chopped
2 garlic cloves, peeled and minced
1 cup onion, peeled and chopped
½ teaspoon Italian seasoning
3 ounces Italian salami, chopped
½ cup Kalamata olives, chopped
4 eggs
½ cup fresh parsley, chopped

Directions:
1.Place squash halves on a lined baking sheet, season with salt and pepper, spread 1 tablespoon butter over them, place in oven at 400ºF, and bake for 45 minutes. Heat a pan with rest of the butter over medium heat, add garlic, onions, salt, and pepper, stir, and cook for a couple of minutes.
2.Add salami and tomatoes, stir, and cook for 10 minutes. Add olives, stir, and cook for a few minutes.
3.Take squash halves out of the oven, scrape flesh with a fork and add with the salami mixture to the pan.
4.Stir, make 4 spaces in the mixture, crack an egg in each, season with salt, pepper, place pan in the oven at 400ºF, and bake until eggs are done. Sprinkle parsley on top and serve.

Nutrition: Calories: 220, Fat: 18.1, Fiber: 1.7, Carbohydrates: 9.4, Protein: 7

Porridge

Prep Time: 5 minutes **Cook Time:** 10 minutes
Servings: 1

Ingredients:
1 teaspoon ground cinnamon
A pinch of nutmeg
½ cup almonds, ground
1 teaspoon stevia
¾ cup coconut cream
A pinch of ground cardamom
A pinch of ground cloves

Directions:
1.Heat a pan over medium heat, add coconut cream, and heat for a few minutes.
2.Add stevia and almonds, stir well, and cook for 5 minutes.
3.Add cloves, cardamom, nutmeg, cinnamon and stir well. Transfer to a bowl and serve hot.

Nutrition: Calories: 695, Fat: 66.7, Fiber: 11.1, Carbohydrates: 22, Protein: 14.3

Nutty Breakfast Bowl

Prep Time: 5 minutes **Cook Time:** 0 minutes
Servings: 1

Ingredients:
1 teaspoon pecans, chopped
½ cup coconut milk
1 teaspoon walnuts, chopped
1 teaspoon pistachios, chopped
1 teaspoon almonds, chopped
1 teaspoon pine nuts, raw
1 teaspoon sunflower seeds, raw
1 teaspoon stevia
2 teaspoons raspberries

Directions:
1.In a bowl, mix milk with honey and stir.
2.Add pecans, walnuts, almonds, pistachios, pine nuts, and sunflower seeds.
3.Stir, top with raspberries, and serve.

Nutrition: Calories: 435, Fat: 44.2, Fiber: 5.2, Carbohydrates: 10.8, Protein: 6.2

Almond Cereal

Prep Time: 5 minutes **Cook Time:** 0 minutes.
Servings: 2

Ingredients:
2 tablespoons almonds, chopped
2 tablespoons sunflower seeds, roasted
⅓ cup coconut milk
1 tablespoon chia seeds
⅓ cup water
½ cup blueberries

Directions:
1.In a bowl, mix chia seeds with coconut milk, and set aside for 5 minutes.
2.In a food processor, mix half of the sunflower seeds with almonds and pulse well.
3.Add this to chia seeds mixture. Add water and stir. Top with rest of the sunflower seeds, blueberries and serve.

Nutrition: Calories: 181, Fat: 15.2, Fiber: 4, Carbohydrates: 10.8, Protein: 3.7

Breakfast Bread

Prep Time: 10 minutes **Cook Time:** 3 minutes
Servings: 4

Ingredients:
½ teaspoon baking powder
⅓ cup almond flour
1 egg, whisked
A pinch of salt
2½ tablespoons coconut oil

Directions:
1.Grease a large microwave–safe mug with some oil. In a bowl, mix egg with flour, salt, oil, and baking powder.
2.Pour into a mug and cook in a microwave for 3 minutes on high.
3.Let the bread cool, take out of the mug, slice, and serve.

Nutrition: Calories: 343, Fat: 38.5, Fiber: 0.4, Carbohydrates: 0.8, Protein: 2.1

Breakfast Muffins

Prep Time: 10 minutes **Cook Time:** 30 minutes
Servings: 4

Ingredients:
½ cup almond milk
6 eggs
1 tablespoon coconut oil
Salt and ground black pepper, to taste
¼ cup kale, chopped
8 prosciutto slices
¼ cup fresh chives, chopped

Directions:
1.In a bowl, mix eggs with salt, pepper, milk, chives, and kale.
2.Grease a muffin tray with melted coconut oil, line with prosciutto slices, pour egg mixture, place in an oven, and bake at 350°F for 30 minutes.
3.Transfer muffins to a platter, and serve.

Nutrition: Calories: 257, Fat: 19.5, Fiber: 0.8, Carbohydrates: 3.4, Protein: 18.1

Vegetable Breakfast Bread

Prep Time: 10 minutes **Cook Time:** 25 minutes
Servings: 7

Ingredients:
1 cauliflower head, separated into florets
½ cup fresh parsley, chopped
1 cup spinach, torn
1 onion, peeled and chopped
1 tablespoon coconut oil
½ cup pecans, ground
3 eggs
2 garlic cloves, peeled and minced
Salt and ground black pepper, to taste

Directions:
1.In a food processor, mix cauliflower florets with some salt, and pepper, and pulse well.
2.Heat a pan with oil over medium heat, add cauliflower, onion, and garlic, some salt and pepper, stir, and cook for 10 minutes. In a bowl, mix eggs with salt, pepper, parsley, spinach, nuts, and stir.
3.Add cauliflower mixture and stir well. Spread mixture into forms placed on a baking sheet, heat oven to 350°F, and bake for 15 minutes. Serve warm.

Nutrition: Calories: 105, Fat: 8.2, Fiber: 2.2, Carbohydrates: 5.2, Protein: 4.2

Breadless Breakfast Sandwich

Prep Time: 10 minutes **Cook Time:** 10 minutes
Servings: 1

Ingredients:
2 eggs
Salt and ground black pepper, to taste
2 tablespoons butter
¼ pound pork sausage, minced
¼ cup water
1 tablespoon guacamole

Directions:
1.In a bowl, mix minced sausage meat with pinch of salt and pepper, and stir well. Shape a patty from mixture and place it on a working surface.
2.Heat a pan with 1 tablespoon butter over medium heat, add sausage patty, fry for 3 minutes on each side, and transfer to a plate.
3.Crack an egg into 2 bowls and whisk with some salt and pepper. Heat a pan with rest of the butter over medium–high heat, place 2 greased biscuit cutters in the pan and add an egg to each.
4.Add water to the pan, reduce heat, cover pan, and cook eggs for 3 minutes. Transfer these egg "buns" to paper towels and drain excess grease.
5.Place sausage patty on one egg "bun," spread guacamole over it, and top with the other egg "bun".

Nutrition: Calories: 735, Fat: 66, Fiber: 0.5, Carbohydrates: 1.7, Protein: 33.6

Granola

Prep Time: 10 minutes **Cook Time:** 0 minutes
Servings: 2

Ingredients:
2 tablespoons chocolate, chopped
7 strawberries, hulled, and chopped
A splash of lemon juice
2 tablespoons pecans, chopped

Directions:
1.In a bowl, mix the chocolate with strawberries, pecans, and lemon juice.
2.Stir well and serve cold.

Nutrition: Calories: 167, Fat: 13.2, Fiber: 2.7, Carbohydrates: 11.5, Protein: 2.6

Chicken Breakfast Muffins

Prep Time: 10 minutes **Cook Time:** 1 hour
Servings: 3

Ingredients:
¾ pound chicken breast, boneless
Salt and ground black pepper, to taste
½ teaspoon garlic powder
1 tbsp cayenne pepper powder mixed with 3 tablespoons melted coconut oil
6 eggs
2 tablespoons green onions, chopped

Directions:
1.Season chicken breast with salt, pepper, and garlic powder, place on a lined baking sheet, and bake in the oven at 425°F for 25 minutes.
2.Transfer chicken breast to a bowl, shred with a fork, and mix with half of the cayenne pepper powder and melted coconut oil. Toss to coat, and set aside.
3.In a bowl, mix eggs with salt, pepper, green onions, and rest of the pepper mixed with oil and whisk.
4.Divide mixture into a muffin tray, top each with shredded chicken, place in oven at 350°F, and bake for 30 minutes. Serve muffins hot.

Nutrition: Calories: 338, Fat: 20.6, Fiber: 0.2, Carbohydrates: 1.3, Protein: 35.3

Turkey Breakfast

Prep Time: 10 minutes **Cook Time:** 20 minutes
Servings: 1

Ingredients:
2 avocado slices
Salt and ground black pepper, to taste
2 bacon slices, diced
2 turkey breast slices, already cooked
2 tablespoons coconut oil
2 eggs, whisked

Directions:
1.Heat a pan over medium heat, add bacon slices, and brown all over.
2.Heat another pan with oil over medium heat, add eggs, salt, pepper, and scramble.
3.Divide turkey breast slices, scrambled eggs, bacon, and avocado slices on 2 plates and serve.

Nutrition: Calories: 791, Fat: 64.3, Fiber: 5.4, Carbohydrates: 11.8, Protein: 41.8

Bacon and Lemon Thyme Muffins

Prep Time: 10 minutes **Cook Time:** 20 minutes
Servings: 12

Ingredients:
1 cup bacon, diced
Salt and ground black pepper, to taste
½ cup butter, melted
3 cups almond flour
1 teaspoon baking soda
4 eggs
2 teaspoons lemon thyme

Directions:
1.In a bowl, mix flour with baking soda, eggs, and stir well. Add butter, lemon thyme, bacon, salt, and pepper, and whisk.
2.Divide mixture into a lined muffin pan, place in an oven at 350°F, and bake for 20 minutes.
3.Let muffins cool, divide on plates, and serve.

Nutrition: Calories: 186, Fat: 17.1, Fiber: 0.8, Carbohydrates: 1.8, Protein: 7.4

Avocado Muffins

Prep Time: 10 minutes **Cook Time:** 20 minutes
Servings: 12

Ingredients:
4 eggs
6 bacon slices, chopped
1 onion, peeled and chopped
1 cup coconut milk
2 cups avocado, pitted, peeled, and chopped
Salt and ground black pepper, to taste
½ teaspoon baking soda
½ cup coconut flour

Directions:
1.Heat a pan over medium heat, add onion, bacon, stir, and cook for a few minutes. In a bowl, mash avocado pieces with a fork and whisk with eggs.
2.Add milk, salt, pepper, baking soda, coconut flour, and stir. Add bacon mixture and stir again.
3.Grease a muffin tray with the coconut oil, divide the eggs and avocado mixture into tray, place in an oven at 350ºF, and bake for 20 minutes.
4.Divide muffins on plates, and serve.

Nutrition: Calories: 175, Fat: 15.1, Fiber: 2.6, Carbohydrates: 4.8, Protein: 6.5

Herbed Biscuits

Prep Time: 10 minutes **Cook Time:** 15 minutes
Servings: 6

Ingredients:
6 tablespoons coconut oil
6 tablespoons coconut flour
2 garlic cloves, peeled and minced
¼ cup onion, minced
2 eggs
Salt and ground black pepper, to taste
1 tablespoons fresh parsley, chopped
2 tablespoons coconut milk
½ teaspoon apple cider vinegar
¼ teaspoon baking soda

Directions:
1.In a bowl, mix coconut flour with eggs, oil, garlic, onion, coconut milk, parsley, salt, pepper, and stir well. In a bowl, mix vinegar with baking soda, stir well, and add to the batter.
2.Drop spoonfuls of batter on lined baking sheets and shape into circles.
3.Place in an oven at 350ºF and bake for 15 minutes. Serve hot.

Nutrition: Calories: 213, Fat: 18.3, Fiber: 5.3, Carbohydrates: 9.2, Protein: 4.1

Naan Bread and Butter

Prep Time: 10 minutes **Cook Time:** 10 minutes
Servings: 6

Ingredients:
7 tablespoons coconut oil
¾ cup coconut flour
2 tablespoons psyllium powder
½ teaspoon baking powder
Salt, to taste
2 cups hot water
Some coconut oil, for frying
2 garlic cloves, peeled and minced
3. 5 ounces butter

Directions:
1.In a bowl, mix coconut flour with baking powder, salt, psyllium powder, and stir. Add coconut oil and the hot water and knead the dough.
2.Set aside for 5 minutes, divide into 6 balls, and flatten them on a working surface.
3.Heat a pan with some coconut oil over medium–high heat, add the naan bread to the pan, fry until golden brown and transfer them to a plate.
4.Heat a pan with the butter over medium–high heat, add garlic, salt, pepper, stir, and cook for 2 minutes.
5.Brush the naan bread with mixture, and pour the rest into a bowl and serve.

Nutrition: Calories: 663, Fat: 73.6, Fiber: 3.6, Carbohydrates: 4.3, Protein: 0.9

Cheese and Oregano Muffins

Prep Time: 10 minutes **Cook Time:** 25 minutes
Servings: 6

Ingredients:

2 tablespoons olive oil
1 egg
2 tablespoons Parmesan cheese
½ teaspoon dried oregano
1 cup almond flour
¼ teaspoon baking soda
Salt and ground black pepper, to taste
½ cup coconut milk
1 cup cheddar cheese, grated

Directions:

1.In a bowl, mix flour with oregano, salt, pepper, Parmesan cheese, and baking soda. In another bowl, mix coconut milk with egg, olive oil, and stir well.
2.Combine the 2 mixtures and whisk.
3.Add cheddar cheese, stir, pour mixture into a lined muffin tray, and place in an oven at 350ºF for 25 minutes.
4.Let muffins cool for a few minutes and serve.

Nutrition: Calories: 204, Fat: 19.1, Fiber: 0.9, Carbohydrates: 2.5, Protein: 7.6

Breakfast Salad in a Jar

Prep Time: 10 minutes **Cook Time:** 0 minutes
Servings: 1

Ingredients:

1 ounce greens
1 ounce red bell pepper, seeded and chopped
1 ounce cherry tomatoes, halved
4 ounces rotisserie chicken, chopped
4 tablespoons extra virgin olive oil
½ scallion, chopped
1 ounce cucumber, chopped
Salt and ground black pepper, to taste

Directions:

1.In a bowl, mix greens with the bell pepper, tomatoes, scallion, cucumber, salt, pepper, olive oil and toss to coat well.
2.Transfer to a jar, top with chicken pieces, and serve.

Nutrition: Calories: 665, Fat: 57.3, Fiber: 3.2, Carbohydrates: 16.1, Protein: 29.8

Lunch

Brussels Sprout Gratin

Prep Time: 10 minutes **Cook Time:** 35 minutes
Servings: 4

Ingredients:
2 ounces onions, diced
1 teaspoon garlic, minced
6 ounces Brussels sprouts, chopped
2 tablespoons butter
1 tablespoon coconut aminos
Salt and ground black pepper, to taste
½ teaspoon liquid smoke
For the sauce:
2. 5 ounces cheddar cheese, grated
A pinch of black pepper
1 tablespoon butter
½ cup heavy cream
¼ teaspoon turmeric
¼ teaspoon paprika
A pinch of xanthan gum
For the pork crust:
3 tablespoons Parmesan cheese
½ ounces pork rinds
½ teaspoon sweet paprika

Directions:
1.Heat a pan with 2 tablespoons butter over high heat, add the Brussels sprouts, salt, pepper, stir, and cook for 3 minutes.
2.Add garlic and onion, stir, and cook for 3 minutes. Add liquid smoke and coconut aminos, stir, take off the heat, and set aside.
3.Heat another pan with 1 tablespoon butter over medium heat, add heavy cream, and stir.
4.Add cheese, black pepper, turmeric, paprika, and xanthan gum, stir, and cook until it thickens again.
5.Add Brussels sprouts mixture, toss to coat, and divide into ramekins.
6.In a food processor, Add the Parmesan cheese with pork rinds, ½ teaspoon paprika, and pulse well.
7.Divide these crumbs on top of Brussels sprouts mixture, place ramekins in the oven at 375ºF, and bake for 20 minutes, and serve.

Nutrition: Calories: 258, Fat: 22.3, Fiber: 2, Carbohydrates: 6.6, Protein: 9.9

Apple Salad

Prep Time: 10 minutes **Cook Time:** 0 minutes
Servings: 4
Ingredients:
2 cups broccoli florets, chopped
2 ounces pecans, chopped
1 apple, cored and grated
1 green onion, diced
Salt and ground black pepper, to taste
2 teaspoons poppy seeds
1 teaspoon apple cider vinegar
¼ cup mayonnaise
½ teaspoon lemon juice
¼ cup sour cream

Directions:
1.In a salad bowl, mix apple with broccoli, green onion, and pecans, and stir.
2.Add poppy seeds, salt, and pepper, and toss gently.
3.In a bowl, mix mayonnaise with sour cream, vinegar, lemon juice, and whisk. Pour over the salad, toss to coat well, and serve cold for lunch.

Nutrition: Calories: 240, Fat: 18.9, Fiber: 4.3, Carbohydrates: 17.5, Protein: 3.9

Caprese Salad

Prep Time: 5 minutes **Cook Time:** 0 minutes
Servings: 2

Ingredients:
½ pound mozzarella cheese, sliced
1 tomato, sliced
Salt and ground black pepper, to taste
4 basil leaves, torn
1 tablespoon balsamic vinegar
1 tablespoon olive oil

Directions:
1.Alternate tomato and mozzarella slices on 2 plates.
2.Sprinkle salt and pepper, drizzle vinegar, and olive oil.
3.Sprinkle with the basil leaves at the end and serve.

Nutrition: Calories: 86, Fat: 8.3, Fiber: 0.4, Carbohydrates: 1.5, Protein: 2.3

Fried Asparagus

Prep Time: 10 minutes **Cook Time:** 10 minutes
Servings: 4

Ingredients:
2 egg yolks
Salt and ground black pepper, to taste
¼ cup butter
1 tablespoon lemon juice
A pinch of cayenne pepper
40 asparagus spears

Directions:
1.In a bowl, whisk the egg yolks well. Transfer to a small pan over low heat.
2.Add lemon juice, and whisk. Add butter and whisk until it melts. Add salt, pepper, cayenne pepper, and whisk again.
3.Heat a pan over medium–high heat, add asparagus spears, and fry them for 5 minutes.
4.Divide asparagus on plates, drizzle with sauce on top, and serve.

Nutrition: Calories: 177, Fat: 14.1, Fiber: 5, Carbohydrates: 9.6, Protein: 6.8

Shrimp Pasta

Prep Time: 10 minutes **Cook Time:** 10 minutes
Servings: 4

Ingredients:
12 ounces Shiritaki noodles
2 tablespoons olive oil
Salt and ground black pepper, to taste
2 tablespoons butter
4 garlic cloves, peeled and minced
1 pound shrimp, peeled and deveined
Juice of ½ lemon
½ teaspoon paprika
½ cup fresh basil, chopped

Directions:
1.Put water in a saucepan, add some salt, bring to a boil, add the Shiritaki noodles, cook for 2 minutes, drain and transfer to a heated pan.
2.Toast the noodles for a few seconds, take off the heat, and leave them aside.
3.Heat a pan with butter and olive oil over medium heat, add the garlic, stir, and brown for 1 minute.
4.Add shrimp, lemon juice, and cook for 3 minutes on each side. Add the noodles, salt, pepper, and paprika, stir, divide into bowls, and serve with chopped basil on top.

Nutrition: Calories: 262, Fat: 15.3, Fiber: 2.2, Carbohydrates: 5.9, Protein: 26.7

Mexican Casserole

Prep Time: 10 minutes **Cook Time:** 35 minutes
Servings: 6

Ingredients:
2 chipotle peppers, chopped
2 jalapeños, chopped
1 tablespoon olive oil
¼ cup heavy cream
1 small white onion, peeled and chopped
Salt and ground black pepper, to taste
1 pound chicken thighs, skinless, boneless, and chopped
1 cup tomato paste
4 ounces cream cheese
Vegetable oil cooking spray
1 cup pepper jack cheese, shredded
2 tablespoons fresh cilantro, chopped
2 homemade tortillas

Directions:
1.Heat a pan with the oil over medium heat, add the chipotle peppers and jalapeño peppers, stir, and cook for a few seconds.
2.Add onion, stir, and cook for 5 minutes. Add cream cheese, heavy cream, and stir until cheese melts.
3.Add chicken, salt, pepper, tomato paste, stir well, and take off the heat.
4.Grease a baking dish with cooking spray, place tortillas on the bottom, spread the chicken mixture all over, and sprinkle with shredded cheese.
5.Cover with aluminum foil, place in an oven at 350ºF, and bake for 15 minutes.
6.Remove the aluminum foil, and bake for 15 minutes. Sprinkle cilantro on top and serve.

Nutrition: Calories: 331, Fat: 19.7, Fiber: 2.4, Carbohydrates: 11.7, Protein: 28.1

Asian Salad

Prep Time: 10 minutes **Cook Time:** 15 minutes
Servings: 4

Ingredients:
1 pound ground beef
2 tablespoons coconut aminos
2 garlic cloves, peeled and minced
2 tablespoon sesame seed oil
1 teaspoon apple cider vinegar
1 teaspoon sesame seeds
1 green onion, chopped

Directions:
1.Heat a pan with the oil over medium heat, add the garlic, and brown for 1 minute. Add beef, stir, and cook for 10 minutes.
2.Make coleslaw mixture, add it into a pan, toss to coat, and cook for 1minute.
3.Add vinegar, sriracha, coconut aminos, salt, pepper, stir, and cook for 4 minutes. Add green onions and sesame seeds, toss to coat, divide into bowls, and serve.

Nutrition: Calories: 281, Fat: 14.3, Fiber: 0.2, Carbohydrates: 1.5, Protein: 34.7

Simple Buffalo Wings

Prep Time: 10 minutes **Cook Time:** 20 minutes
Servings: 2

Ingredients:
2 tablespoons butter
6 chicken wings, cut in half
Salt and ground black pepper, to taste
A pinch of garlic powder
3 tbsp cayenne pepper powder
4 tbsp olive oil
A pinch of cayenne pepper
½ teaspoon sweet paprika

Directions:
1.In a bowl, mix chicken pieces with half of the hot sauce, salt, and pepper, and toss well to coat.
2.Arrange chicken pieces on a lined baking dish, place under a preheated broiler, and broil 8 minutes. Flip chicken pieces, and broil for 8 minutes.
3.Heat a pan with the butter over medium heat. Add the rest of the hot sauce, salt, pepper, cayenne, and paprika, stir, and cook for a couple of minutes.
4.Transfer broiled chicken pieces to a bowl, add the butter, and pour olive oil and cayenne pepper mixture over them, toss to coat well, and serve.

Nutrition: Calories: 610, Fat: 50, Fiber: 0.2, Carbohydrates: 0.4, Protein: 40.7

Bacon and Mushroom Skewers

Prep Time: 10 minutes **Cook Time:** 20 minutes
Servings: 6

Ingredients:
1 pound mushroom caps
6 bacon strips
Salt and ground black pepper, to taste
½ teaspoon sweet paprika
Sweet mesquite seasoning

Directions:
1.Season the mushroom caps with salt, pepper, and paprika.
2.Spear a bacon strip on a skewer. Spear a mushroom cap, and fold the bacon over it. Repeat until you obtain a mushroom and bacon braid.
3.Repeat with the rest of the mushrooms and bacon strips.
4.Season with sweet mesquite, place all skewers on a preheated kitchen grill over medium heat, cook for 10 minutes, flip, and cook for 10 minutes. Divide on plates and serve.

Nutrition: Calories: 47, Fat: 2.9, Fiber: 0.8, Carbohydrates: 2.6, Protein: 3.6

Simple Tomato Soup

Prep Time: 10 minutes **Cook Time:** 5 minutes
Servings: 4

Ingredients:
1 quart canned tomato passata
4 tablespoons butter
½ cup olive oil
3 tbsp cayenne pepper powder
2 tablespoons apple cider vinegar
Salt and ground black pepper, to taste
1 teaspoon dried oregano
2 teaspoons turmeric
8 bacon strips, cooked and crumbled
½ cup green onions, chopped
½ cup fresh basil leaves, chopped

Directions:
1.Put the tomato passata in a saucepan and heat over medium.
2.Add olive oil, butter, cayenne pepper, vinegar, salt, pepper, turmeric, oregano, stir, and simmer for 5 minutes.
3.Take off heat, divide soup into bowls, top with crumbled bacon, basil, and green onions.

Nutrition: Calories: 385, Fat: 41.4, Fiber: 0.8, Carbohydrates: 3.5, Protein: 2.9

Bacon–wrapped Sausages

Prep Time: 10 minutes **Cook Time:** 30 minutes
Servings: 4

Ingredients:
8 bacon strips
8 sausages
16 pepper jack cheese slices
Salt and ground black pepper, to taste
A pinch of garlic powder
½ teaspoon sweet paprika
1 pinch of onion powder

Directions:
1.Heat a kitchen grill over medium heat, add the sausages, cook for a few minutes on each side, transfer to a plate, and set aside for a few minutes to cool down.
2.Cut a slit in the middle of each sausage to create pockets, stuff each with 2 cheese slices, and season with salt, pepper, paprika, onion, and garlic powder.
3.Wrap each stuffed sausage in a bacon strip, secure with toothpicks, place on a lined baking sheet, place in an oven at 400ºF, bake for 15 minutes, and serve.

Nutrition: Calories: 501, Fat: 41.8, Fiber: 0, Carbohydrates: 0, Protein: 49.6

Lobster Bisque

Prep Time: 10 minutes **Cook Time:** 1 hour
Servings: 4

Ingredients:
4 garlic cloves, peeled and minced
1 onion, peeled and chopped
24 ounces lobster chunks, precooked
Salt and ground black pepper, to taste
½ cup tomato paste
5 oz butternut squash, diced
4 celery stalks, chopped
1–quart seafood stock
1 tablespoon olive oil
1 cup heavy cream
3 bay leaves
1 teaspoon dried thyme
1 teaspoon peppercorns
1 teaspoon paprika
1 teaspoon xanthan gum
½ cup fresh parsley, chopped
1 tablespoon lemon juice

Directions:
1.Heat a pot with oil over medium heat, add onion, stir, and cook for 4 minutes.
2.Add garlic, stir, and cook for 1 minute. Add celery and squash, stir, and cook for 1 minute. Add tomato paste, and stock, and stir.
3.Add bay leaves, salt, pepper, peppercorns, paprika, thyme, and xanthan gum, stir, and simmer over medium heat for 1 hour.
4.Discard bay leaves, add the cream, and bring to a simmer. Blend using an immersion blender, add lobster chunks, and cook for a few minutes.
5.Add lemon juice, stir, divide into bowls, and sprinkle parsley on top.

Nutrition: Calories: 359, Fat: 16.8, Fiber: 5, Carbohydrates: 33.2, Protein: 20.7

Beef Shank Stew

Prep Time: 10 minutes **Cook Time:** 3 hours and 30 minutes
Servings: 6

Ingredients:
8 tomatoes, cored and chopped
5 pounds beef shanks
6 oz butternut squash, peeled and chopped
8 garlic cloves, peeled and minced
2 onions, peeled and chopped
2 cups water
1–quart chicken stock
¼ cup tomato sauce
Salt and ground black pepper, to taste
2 tablespoons apple cider vinegar
3 bay leaves
3 teaspoons red pepper, crushed
2 teaspoons dried parsley
2 teaspoons dried basil
2 teaspoons garlic powder
2 teaspoons onion powder
A pinch of cayenne pepper

Directions:
1.Heat a pot over medium heat, add garlic, squash, onions, stir, and brown for a few minutes.
2.Heat a pan over medium heat, add beef shank, brown for a few minutes on each side, and take off heat.
3.Add stock over squash, water, vinegar, and stir.
4.Add tomatoes, tomato sauce, salt, pepper, cayenne pepper, crushed pepper, bay leaves, basil, parsley, onion powder, garlic powder, and stir.
5.Add beef shanks, cover pot, bring to a simmer, and cook for 3 hours.
6.Discard the bay leaves, divide into bowls, and serve.

Nutrition: Calories: 832, Fat: 24.9, Fiber: 3.6, Carbohydrates: 15.5, Protein: 130.3

Chicken and Shrimp

Prep Time: 10 minutes **Cook Time:** 20 minutes
Servings: 2

Ingredients:
20 shrimp, raw, peeled, and deveined
2 chicken breasts, boneless, and skinless
2 handfuls spinach leaves
½ pound mushrooms, chopped
Salt and ground black pepper, to taste
¼ cup mayonnaise
2 tablespoons sriracha
2 teaspoons lime juice
1 tablespoon coconut oil
½ teaspoon red pepper, crushed
1 teaspoon garlic powder
½ teaspoon paprika
¼ teaspoon xanthan gum
1 green onion, chopped

Directions:
1.Heat a pan with the oil over medium–high heat, add chicken breasts, season with salt, pepper, red pepper, garlic powder, cook for 8 minutes, flip, and cook for 6 minutes.
2.Add mushrooms, more salt and pepper, and cook for a few minutes.
3.Heat another pan over medium heat, add shrimp, sriracha, paprika, xanthan, mayonnaise, stir, and cook until shrimp turns pink. Take off heat, add lime juice, and stir.
4.Divide spinach on plates, add chicken and mushroom, top with shrimp mixture, garnish with green onions, and serve.

Nutrition: Calories: 1052, Fat: 42.5, Fiber: 3.1, Carbohydrates: 22.2, Protein: 140.2

Green Soup

Prep Time: 10 minutes **Cook Time:** 13 minutes
Servings: 6

Ingredients:
1 cauliflower head, separated into florets
1 white onion, peeled and diced
1 bay leaf, crushed
2 garlic cloves, peeled and minced
5 ounces watercress
7 ounces spinach leaves
1quart vegetable stock
1 cup coconut milk
Salt and ground black pepper, to taste
¼ cup butter
½ cup parsley, for serving

Directions:
1.Heat a pot with the butter over medium–high heat, add garlic, and onion, stir, and brown for 4 minutes.
2.Add cauliflower and bay leaf, stir, and cook for 5 minutes. Add watercress and spinach, stir, and cook for 3 minutes.
3.Add stock, salt, pepper, stir, and bring to a boil.
4.Add coconut milk, stir, take off heat, and blend using an immersion blender. Divide into bowls and serve.

Nutrition: Calories: 194, Fat: 17.6, Fiber: 3.6, Carbohydrates: 8.2, Protein: 3.9

Salmon Soup

Prep Time: 10 minutes **Cook Time:** 25 minutes
Servings: 4

Ingredients:
4 leeks, trimmed, and sliced
Salt and ground black pepper, to taste
2 tablespoons avocado oil
2 garlic cloves, peeled and minced
6 cups chicken stock
1 pound salmon, cut into small pieces
2 teaspoons dried thyme
1¾ cups coconut milk

Directions:
1.Heat a pot with the oil over medium heat, add the leeks and garlic, stir, and cook for 5 minutes.
2.Add thyme, stock, salt, and pepper, stir, and simmer for 15 minutes.
3.Add coconut milk, salmon, stir, and bring to a simmer again. Divide into bowls and serve.

Nutrition: Calories: 680, Fat: 55.5, Fiber: 6.4, Carbohydrates: 25.7, Protein: 29.1

Halloumi Salad

Prep Time: 10 minutes **Cook Time:** 10 minutes
Servings: 1

Ingredients:
3 ounces halloumi cheese, sliced
1 cucumber, sliced
1 ounce walnuts, chopped
A drizzle of olive oil
½ cup baby arugula
5 cherry tomatoes, halved
A splash of balsamic vinegar
Salt and ground black pepper, to taste

Directions:
1.Heat a kitchen grill over medium–high heat, add halloumi pieces, grill them for 5 minutes on each side, and transfer to a plate.
2.In a bowl, mix tomatoes with cucumber, walnuts, and arugula.
3.Add halloumi pieces on top, season everything with salt, pepper, drizzle the oil, and the vinegar, toss to coat, and serve.

Nutrition: Calories: 643, Fat: 43.7, Fiber: 11, Carbohydrates: 40.2, Protein: 32.8

Halibut Soup

Prep Time: 10 minutes **Cook Time:** 30 minutes
Servings: 4

Ingredients:
1 onion, peeled and chopped
1 pound butternut squash, peeled and sliced
1 tablespoon coconut oil
Salt and ground black pepper, to taste
2 tablespoons ginger, minced
1 cup water
1 pound halibut, cut into medium chunks
12 cups chicken stock

Directions:
1.Heat a pot with the oil over medium heat, add the onion, stir, and cook for 6 minutes. Add ginger, squash, water, and stock, stir and bring to a simmer.
2.Reduce temperature, and cook for 20 minutes. Blend the soup using an immersion blender, season with salt and pepper, and add the halibut pieces.
3.Stir gently and simmer soup for 5 minutes. Divide into bowls and serve.

Nutrition: Calories: 240, Fat: 7.4, Fiber: 3.2, Carbohydrates: 19.9, Protein: 26.7

Cauliflower Mash

Prep Time: 10 minutes **Cook Time:** 10 minutes
Servings: 2

Ingredients:
¼ cup sour cream
1 small cauliflower head, separated into florets
Salt and ground black pepper, to taste
2 tablespoons feta cheese, crumbled
2 tablespoons black olives, pitted and sliced

Directions:
1.Put water in a saucepan, add some salt, bring to a boil over medium heat, add the florets, cook for 10 minutes, take off heat, and drain.
2.Return cauliflower to the saucepan, add salt, black pepper, and sour cream, and blend using an immersion blender.
3.Add black olives and feta cheese, stir, and serve.

Nutrition: Calories: 129, Fat: 9.1, Fiber: 3.6, Carbohydrates: 9.2, Protein: 4.9

Portobello Mushrooms

Prep Time: 10 minutes **Cook Time:** 10 minutes
Servings: 4

Ingredients:
12 ounces Portobello mushrooms, sliced
Salt and ground black pepper, to taste
½ teaspoon dried basil
2 tablespoons olive oil
½ teaspoon tarragon, dried
½ teaspoon dried rosemary
½ teaspoon dried thyme
2 tablespoons balsamic vinegar

Directions:
1.In a bowl, mix the oil with vinegar, salt, pepper, rosemary, tarragon, basil, and thyme, and whisk.
2.Add mushroom slices, toss to coat well, place them on a preheated grill over medium–high heat, cook for 5 minutes on both sides, and serve.

Nutrition: Calories: 85, Fat: 7, Fiber: 0, Carbohydrates: 2.5, Protein: 2.5

Brussels Sprouts and Bacon

Prep Time: 10 minutes **Cook Time:** 30 minutes **Servings:** 4

Ingredients:
8 bacon strips, chopped
1 pound Brussels sprouts, trimmed, and halved
Salt and ground black pepper, to taste
A pinch of cumin
A pinch of red pepper, crushed
2 tablespoons extra virgin olive oil

Directions:
1.In a bowl, mix Brussels sprouts with salt, pepper, cumin, red pepper, and oil, and toss to coat.
2.Spread Brussels sprouts on a lined baking sheet, place in an oven at 375°F, and bake for 30 minutes.
3.Heat a pan over medium heat, add bacon pieces, and cook them until crispy. Divide the baked Brussels sprouts on plates, top with bacon, and serve.

Nutrition: Calories: 159, Fat: 11.9, Fiber: 4.3, Carbohydrates: 10.3, Protein: 5.9

Ketogenic Side Dish Recipes Simple Kimchi

Prep Time: 1 hour and 10 minutes **Cook Time:** 0 minutes **Servings:** 6

Ingredients:
3 tablespoons salt
1 pound napa cabbage, chopped
3 oz butternut squash, julienned
½ cup daikon radish
3 green onion stalks, chopped
1 tablespoon fish sauce
3 tablespoons chili flakes
3 garlic cloves, peeled and minced
1 tablespoon sesame oil
½–inchfresh ginger, peeled and grated

Directions:
1.In a bowl, mix cabbage with salt, massage well for 10 minutes, cover, and set aside for 1 hour.
2.In a bowl, mix the chili flakes with fish sauce, garlic, sesame oil, ginger, and stir well.
3.Drain cabbage well, rinse under cold water, and transfer to a bowl.
4.Add squash, green onions, radish, and chili paste, and stir. Leave in a dark and cold place for at least 2 days before serving.

Nutrition: Calories: 43, Fat: 2.5, Fiber: 1.5, Carbohydrates: 4.9, Protein: 1.6

Oven–fried Green Beans

Prep Time: 10 minutes **Cook Time:** 10 minutes **Servings:** 4

Ingredients:
⅔ cup Parmesan cheese, grated
1 egg
12 ounces green beans
Salt and ground black pepper, to taste
½ teaspoon garlic powder
¼ teaspoon paprika

Directions:
1.In a bowl, mix Parmesan cheese with salt, pepper, garlic powder, and paprika. In another bowl, whisk egg with salt and pepper.
2.Coat the green beans in egg, and then in the Parmesan mixture.
3.Place green beans on a lined baking sheet, place in an oven at 400°F for 10 minutes. Serve hot.

Nutrition: Calories: 66, Fat: 2.7, Fiber: 3, Carbohydrates: 6.7, Protein: 5.3

Broiled Brussels Sprouts

Prep Time: 10 minutes **Cook Time:** 10 minutes
Servings: 4

Ingredients:
1 pound Brussels sprouts, trimmed, and halved
Salt and ground black pepper, to taste
1 teaspoon sesame seeds
1 tablespoon green onions, chopped
1½ tablespoons sukrin gold syrup
1 tablespoon coconut aminos
2 tablespoons sesame oil
1 tablespoon sriracha

Directions:
1.In a bowl, mix the sesame oil with coconut aminos, sriracha, syrup, salt, and black pepper, and whisk.
2.Heat a pan over medium–high heat, add the Brussels sprouts, and cook them for 5 minutes on each side.
3.Add the sesame oil mixture, toss to coat, sprinkle sesame seeds, green onions, stir again, and serve.

Nutrition: Calories: 192, Fat: 7.6, Fiber: 4.4, Carbohydrates: 30.3, Protein: 4

Pesto

Prep Time: 10 minutes **Cook Time:** 0 minutes
Servings: 4

Ingredients:
½ cup olive oil
2 cups basil
⅓ cup pine nuts
⅓ cup Parmesan cheese, grated
2 garlic cloves, peeled and chopped
Salt and ground black pepper, to taste

Directions:
1.Put basil in a food processor, add pine nuts, garlic, and blend well.
2.Add the Parmesan cheese, salt, pepper, and the oil gradually and blend again until you obtain a paste. Serve with chicken or vegetables.

Nutrition: Calories: 320, Fat: 34.5, Fiber: 0.6, Carbohydrates: 2.6, Protein: 4.3

Creamy Spinach

Prep Time: 10 minutes **Cook Time:** 15 minutes
Servings: 2

Ingredients:
2 garlic cloves, peeled and minced
8 ounces spinach leaves
A drizzle of olive oil
Salt and ground black pepper, to taste
4 tablespoons sour cream
1 tablespoon butter
2 tablespoons Parmesan cheese, grated

Directions:
1.Heat a pan with the oil over medium heat, add spinach, stir and cook until it softens.
2.Add salt, pepper, butter, Parmesan cheese, stir and cook for 4 minutes.
3.Add sour cream, stir, and cook for 5 minutes. Divide on plates and serve.

Nutrition: Calories: 144, Fat: 12, Fiber: 2.6, Carbohydrates: 6.3, Protein: 5.4

Avocado Fries

Prep Time: 10 minutes **Cook Time:** 5 minutes
Servings: 3

Ingredients:
3 avocados, pitted, peeled, halved, and sliced
1½ cups sunflower oil
1½ cups almond meal
A pinch of cayenne pepper
Salt and ground black pepper, to taste

Directions:
1.In a bowl, mix almond meal with salt, pepper, cayenne, and stir. In a second bowl, whisk eggs with a pinch of salt and pepper.
2.Coat the avocado pieces in egg, and then in almond meal mixture.
3.Heat a pan with oil over medium–high heat, add avocado fries, and cook them until they are golden.
4.Transfer to paper towels, drain grease, and divide on plates and serve.

Nutrition: Calories: 1648, Fat: 172, Fiber: 19.4, Carbohydrates: 27.5, Protein: 13.9

Okra and Tomatoes

Prep Time: 10 minutes **Cook Time:** 10 minutes
Servings: 6

Ingredients:
14 ounces canned stewed tomatoes, cored and chopped
Salt and ground black pepper, to taste
2 celery stalks, chopped
1 onion, peeled and chopped
1 pound okra, trimmed and sliced
2 bacon slices, chopped
1 small green bell peppers, seeded and chopped

Directions:
1.Heat a pan over medium–high heat, add bacon, stir, brown for a few minutes, transfer to paper towels, and set aside.
2.Heat the pan again over medium heat, add okra, bell pepper, onion, and celery, stir, and cook for 2 minutes.
3.Add tomatoes, salt, and pepper, stir, and cook for 3 minutes. Divide on plates, garnish with crispy bacon, and serve.

Nutrition: Calories: 91, Fat: 3, Fiber: 14, Carbohydrates: 11.7, Protein: 4.7

Mushroom Salad

Prep Time: 10 minutes **Cook Time:** 10 minutes
Servings: 4

Ingredients:
2 tablespoons butter
1 pound cremini mushrooms, chopped
4 tablespoons extra virgin olive oil
Salt and ground black pepper, to taste
4 bunches arugula
8 slices prosciutto
2 tablespoons apple cider vinegar
8 sundried tomatoes in oil, drained, and chopped
Parmesan cheese, shaved
Fresh parsley leaves, chopped

Directions:
1.Heat a pan with butter and half of the oil over medium–high heat.
2.Add mushrooms, salt, and pepper, stir, and cook for 3 minutes. Reduce heat, stir again, and cook for 3 more minutes.
3.Add rest of the oil and vinegar, stir and cook 1 minute.
4.Place arugula on a serving platter, add prosciutto on top, add the mushroom mixture, sundried tomatoes, more salt and pepper, Parmesan shavings, parsley, and serve.

Nutrition: Calories: 352, Fat: 24.8, Fiber: 2.4, Carbohydrates: 15.5, Protein: 16.3

Collard Greens with Turkey

Prep Time: 10 minutes **Cook Time:** 2 hours and 15 minutes
Servings: 10

Ingredients:
5 bunches collard greens, chopped
Salt and ground black pepper, to taste
1 tablespoon red pepper flakes
5 cups chicken stock
1 turkey leg
2 tablespoons garlic, minced
¼ cup olive oil

Directions:
1.Heat a pot with the oil over medium heat, add garlic, stir, and cook for 1 minute. Add stock, salt, pepper, turkey leg, stir, cover, and simmer for 30 minutes.
2.Add collard greens, cover pot again, and cook for 45 minutes.
3.Reduce heat to medium, add more salt and pepper, stir, and cook for 1 hour.
4.Drain the greens, chop up the turkey, mix everything with the red pepper flakes, stir, divide on plates, and serve.

Nutrition: Calories: 171, Fat: 10.9, Fiber: 0.8, Carbohydrates: 2.2, Protein: 16.1

Edamame and Mint

Prep Time: 10 minutes **Cook Time:** 5 minutes
Servings: 4

Ingredients:
¾ pound edamame
Salt and ground black pepper, to taste
1 tablespoon mint leaves, chopped
2 teaspoons olive oil
3 green onions, chopped
1 garlic clove, peeled and minced

Directions:
1.Heat a pan with the oil over medium–high heat. Add edamame, salt, pepper, green onions, garlic, and mint.
2.Stir everything, cook for 5 minutes, divide on plates, and serve.

Nutrition: Calories: 91, Fat: 3, Fiber: 4, Carbohydrates: 11.7, Protein: 4.7

Eggplant and Tomatoes

Prep Time: 10 minutes **Cook Time:** 15 minutes
Servings: 4

Ingredients:
1 tomato, sliced
1 eggplant, sliced into thin rounds
Salt and ground black pepper, to taste
¼ cup Parmesan cheese, grated
A drizzle of olive oil

Directions:
1.Place eggplant slices on a lined baking dish, drizzle some oil, and sprinkle half of the Parmesan.
2.Top eggplant slices with tomato ones, season with some salt and pepper, and sprinkle the rest of the cheese over them.
3.Place in an oven at 400ºF, and bake for 15 minutes. Divide on plates and serve hot as a side dish.

Nutrition: Calories: 73, Fat: 4.5, Fiber: 4.5, Carbohydrates: 7.2, Protein: 2.4

Sautéed Broccoli

Prep Time: 10 minutes **Cook Time:** 22 minutes
Servings: 4

Ingredients:
5 tablespoons olive oil
1 garlic clove, peeled and minced
1 pound broccoli florets
1 tablespoon Parmesan cheese, grated
Salt and ground black pepper, to taste

Directions:
1.Put water in a saucepan, add salt, bring to a boil over medium–high heat, add broccoli, cook for 5 minutes, and drain.
2.Heat a pan with oil over medium–high heat, add garlic, stir, and cook for 2 minutes. Add broccoli, stir, and cook for 15 minutes.
3.Take off heat, sprinkle Parmesan cheese, divide on plates, and serve.

Nutrition: Calories: 195, Fat: 18.2, Fiber: 3, Carbohydrates: 7.8, Protein: 3.8

Easy Grilled Onions

Prep Time: 10 minutes **Cook Time:** 1 hour
Servings: 4

Ingredients:
½ cup butter
4 onions
4 chicken bouillon cubes
Salt and ground black pepper, to taste

Direction:
1.Cut the onion tops and make a hole in the middle, divide the butter and chicken bouillon cubes into these holes, and season with salt and pepper.
2.Wrap onions in aluminum foil, place them on preheated kitchen grill, and grill for 1 hour.
3.Unwrap the onions, chop them into big chunks, arrange on plates, and serve.

Nutrition: Calories: 256, Fat: 23.5, Fiber: 2.4, Carbohydrates: 11.1, Protein: 2

Sautéed Zucchini

Prep Time: 10 minutes **Cook Time:** 15 minutes
Servings: 6

Ingredients:
1 onion, peeled and chopped
1 tomato, cored and chopped
½ pound tomatoes, cored and chopped
Salt and ground black pepper, to taste
1 garlic clove, peeled and minced
1 teaspoon Italian seasoning
4 zucchini, sliced

Directions:
1.Heat a pan with oil over medium heat, add onion, salt, pepper, stir, and cook for 2 minutes.
2.Add mushrooms, zucchini, stir, and cook for 5 minutes. Add garlic, tomatoes, Italian seasoning, stir, cook for 6 minutes.
3.Take off heat, divide on plates, and serve.

Nutrition: Calories: 42, Fat: 0.6, Fiber: 2.6, Carbohydrates: 8.7, Protein: 2.4

Greek Side Salad

Prep Time: 10 minutes **Cook Time:** 7 minutes
Servings: 6

Ingredients:
½ pounds mushrooms, sliced
1 tablespoon extra virgin olive oil
3 garlic cloves, peeled and minced
1 teaspoon dried basil
Salt and ground black pepper, to taste
1 tomato, cored and diced
3 tablespoons lemon juice
½ cup water
1 tablespoons coriander, chopped

Directions:
1.Heat a pan with the oil over medium heat, add mushrooms, stir, and cook for 3 minutes.
2.Add basil and garlic, stir, and cook for 1 minute. Add water, salt, pepper, tomato, and lemon juice, stir, and cook for a few minutes.
3.Take off heat, transfer to a bowl, set aside to cool down, sprinkle the coriander, and serve.

Nutrition: Calories: 34, Fat: 2.5, Fiber: 0.6, Carbohydrates: 2.3, Protein: 1.4

Fried Swiss Chard

Prep Time: 10 minutes **Cook Time:** 10 minutes
Servings: 2

Ingredients:
2 tablespoons butter
4 bacon slices, chopped
1 bunch Swiss chard, chopped
½ teaspoon garlic paste
3 tablespoons lemon juice
Salt and ground black pepper, to taste

Directions:
1.Heat a pan over medium heat, add bacon pieces, and cook until crispy.
2.Add butter, and stir until it melts. Add garlic paste and lemon juice, stir, and cook for 1 minute.
3.Add Swiss chard, stir, and cook for 4 minutes.
4.Add salt and black pepper to taste, stir, divide on plates, and serve.

Nutrition: Calories: 317, Fat: 27.6, Fiber: 0.4, Carbohydrates: 1.9, Protein: 14.7

Tomato Salsa

Prep Time: 2 hours **Cook Time:** 0 minutes
Servings: 5

Ingredients:
3 yellow tomatoes, seeded and chopped
1 red tomato, seeded and chopped
Salt and ground black pepper, to taste
⅓ cup onion, diced
2 jalapeño peppers, diced
¼ cup cilantro, diced
3 tablespoons lime juice
1/3 teaspoons stevia

Directions:
1.In a bowl, mix tomatoes with onion, and jalapeño.
2.Add cilantro, lime juice, salt, pepper, stevia, and stir well.
3.Cover the bowl, keep in the refrigerator for 2 hours, and serve.

Nutrition: Calories: 24, Fat: 0.4, Fiber: 1.2, Carbohydrates: 5.2, Protein: 1.3

Summer Side Salad

Prep Time: 10 minutes **Cook Time:** 5 minutes
Servings: 6

Ingredients:
½ cup extra virgin olive oil
1 cucumber, chopped
2 pints colored cherry tomatoes, cut into half
Salt and ground black pepper, to taste
1 onion, peeled and chopped
3 tablespoons balsamic vinegar
1 garlic clove, peeled and minced
1 bunch fresh basil, chopped

Directions:
1.In a bowl, mix vinegar with salt, pepper, and olive oil and whisk. In a salad bowl, mix the cucumber with tomatoes, onion, garlic.
2.Add vinegar dressing, toss to coat, sprinkle the basil, add more salt and pepper, if needed, toss to coat, and serve.

Nutrition: Calories: 171, Fat: 17, Fiber: 1.3, Carbohydrates: 5.8, Protein: 1.3

Cucumber and Cashew Salad

Prep Time: 10 minutes **Cook Time:** 0 minutes
Servings: 4

Ingredients:
2 English cucumbers, chopped
4 oz cashews, crushed
¾ cup fennel, sliced thin
2 tablespoons fresh chives, diced
½ cup walnuts, chopped
2 tablespoons lemon juice
4 tablespoons fruity olive oil
Salt and ground black pepper, to taste

Directions:
1.Put cucumber on a paper towel, press well, and transfer to a salad bowl. Crush slightly with a fork.
2.Add cashews, fennel, chives, walnuts, and stir gently.
3.Add salt, pepper, lemon juice, and the oil, toss to coat, and serve.

Nutrition: Calories: 407, Fat: 36.6, Fiber: 3.2, Carbohydrates: 17.5, Protein: 9.3

Tomato and Bocconcini

Prep Time: 6 minutes **Cook Time:** 0 minutes
Servings: 4

Ingredients:
20 ounces tomatoes, cut in wedges
2 tablespoons extra virgin olive oil
1½ tablespoons balsamic vinegar
1 teaspoon stevia
1 garlic clove, minced
8 ounces baby bocconcini, drained and torn
1 cup fresh basil leaves, chopped
Salt and ground black pepper, to taste

Directions:
1.In a bowl, mix stevia with vinegar, garlic, oil, salt, and pepper, and whisk.
2.In a salad bowl, mix bocconcini with the tomato and basil. Add the dressing, toss to coat, and serve.

Nutrition: Calories: 332, Fat: 29.3, Fiber: 1.8, Carbohydrates: 8.1, Protein: 11.5

Indian Mint Chutney

Prep Time: 10 minutes **Cook Time:** 0 minutes
Servings: 8

Ingredients:
1½ cup mint leaves
1 bunch cilantro, stems removed
Salt and ground black pepper, to taste
1 green chili pepper, seedless
1 onion, cut into medium–sized chunks
¼ cup water
1 tablespoon tamarind juice

Directions:
1.Put mint and cilantro leaves in a food processor and blend.
2.Add the chili pepper, salt, black pepper, onion, and tamarind paste and blend again.
3.Add water, blend again until you obtain cream, transfer to a bowl, and serve.

Nutrition: Calories: 36, Fat: 0.5, Fiber: 4.7, Carbohydrates: 7.3, Protein: 2.3

Broccoli with Lemon Almond Butter

Prep Time: 10 minutes **Cook Time:** 10 minutes
Servings: 4

Ingredients:
1 broccoli head, separated into florets
Salt and ground black pepper, to taste
¼ cup almonds, blanched
1 teaspoon lemon zest
¼ cup coconut butter, melted
2 tablespoons lemon juice

Directions:
1.Put water in a saucepan, add the salt, and bring to a boil over medium–high heat.
2.Place broccoli florets in a steamer basket, place into saucepan, cover, and steam for 8 minutes. Drain and transfer to a bowl.
3.Heat a pan with the coconut butter over medium heat, add the lemon juice, lemon zest, and almonds, stir, and take off heat.
4.Add the broccoli, toss to coat, divide on plates, and serve.

Nutrition: Calories: 168, Fat: 12.4, Fiber: 6.3, Carbohydrates: 12.6, Protein: 5.5

Eggplant Salad

Prep Time: 10 minutes **Cook Time:** 10 minutes
Servings: 4

Ingredients:
1 eggplant, sliced
1 onion, peeled and sliced
A drizzle of canola oil
1 avocado, pitted and chopped
1 teaspoon mustard
1 tablespoon balsamic vinegar
1 tablespoon fresh oregano, chopped
A drizzle of olive oil
Salt and ground black pepper, to taste
Zest from 1 lemon
Fresh parsley, chopped, for serving

Directions:
1.Brush onion and eggplant slices with a drizzle of canola oil, place them on a heated kitchen grill, and cook until they become soft.
2.Transfer to a cutting board, leave to cool down, chop, and put in a bowl. Add avocado and stir gently.
3.In a bowl, mix vinegar with mustard, oregano, olive oil, salt and pepper to taste.
4.Add this to the eggplant, avocado, and onion mixture, toss to coat, add the lemon zest and parsley on top, and serve.

Nutrition: Calories: 181, Fat: 13.9, Fiber: 8.6, Carbohydrates: 14.7, Protein: 2.7

Baked Eggplant Side Salad

Prep Time: 2 hours and 10 minutes **Cook Time:** 1 hour and 30 minutes
Servings: 12

Ingredients:
1 garlic clove, peeled and crushed
6 eggplants
1 teaspoon dried parsley
1 teaspoon dried oregano
¼ teaspoon dried basil
3 tablespoons extra virgin olive oil
2 tablespoons stevia
1 tablespoon balsamic vinegar
Salt and ground black pepper, to taste

Directions:
1.Prick eggplants with a fork, arrange on a baking sheet, place in an oven at 350ºF and bake for 1 hour and 30 minutes.
2.Take out of the oven, leave them to cool down, peel, chop, and transfer to a salad bowl.
3.Add garlic, oil, parsley, stevia, oregano, basil, salt, pepper, toss to coat, keep in the refrigerator for 2 hours, and then serve.

Nutrition: Calories: 100, Fat: 4, Fiber: 9.7, Carbohydrates: 16.3, Protein: 2.7

Endive and Watercress Side Salad

Prep Time: 10 minutes **Cook Time:** 5 minutes
Servings: 4

Ingredients:
4 medium endives, roots and ends cut and sliced thin crosswise
1 tablespoon lemon juice
1 shallot, peeled and diced
1 tablespoon balsamic vinegar
2 tablespoons extra virgin olive oil
6 tablespoons heavy cream
Salt and ground black pepper, to taste
4 ounces watercress, chopped
1 tablespoon fresh chervil, chopped
1 tablespoon fresh tarragon, chopped
1 tablespoon fresh chives, chopped
⅓ cup almonds, chopped
1 tablespoon fresh parsley, chopped

Directions:
1.In a bowl, mix lemon juice with vinegar, salt, and shallot, stir, and set aside for 10 minutes. Add olive oil, pepper, stir, and set aside for 2 minutes.
2.Put endives, watercress, chives, tarragon, parsley, and chervil in a salad bowl. Add salt and pepper to taste and toss to coat.
3.Add heavy cream and vinaigrette, stir gently, and serve with almonds on top.

Nutrition: Calories: 204, Fat: 19.6, Fiber: 2.3, Carbohydrates: 5.2, Protein: 3.8

Indian Side Salad

Prep Time: 15 minutes **Cook Time:** 0 minutes
Servings: 6

Ingredients:
7 oz butternut squash, peeled and grated
2 zucchini, sliced thin
A bunch of radishes, finely sliced
½ onion, peeled and chopped
6 mint leaves, chopped
For the salad dressing:
1 teaspoon mustard
1 tablespoon homemade mayo
1 tablespoon balsamic vinegar
2 tablespoons extra virgin olive oil
Salt and ground black pepper, to taste

Directions:
1.In a bowl, mix mustard with mayonnaise, vinegar, salt, and pepper, and stir well. Add oil gradually and whisk.
2.In a salad bowl, mix squash with radishes, zucchini, and mint leaves.
3.Add the salad dressing, toss to coat, and keep in the refrigerator until ready to serve.

Nutrition: Calories: 71, Fat: 4.8, Fiber: 1.8, Carbohydrates: 7.3, Protein: 1.3

Indian Coconut Chutney

Prep Time: 5 minutes **Cook Time:** 5 minutes
Servings: 3

Ingredients:
½ teaspoon cumin
½ cup coconut, grated
2 tablespoons chana dal, already fried
2 green chilies
Salt, to taste
1 garlic clove, peeled
¾ tablespoons avocado oil
¼ teaspoon mustard seeds
A pinch of hing
½ teaspoons urad dal
1 red chili chopped
1 spring curry leaves

Directions:
1.In a food processor, mix coconut with salt, cumin, garlic, chana dal, green chilies and blend well. Add a splash of water, blend again.
2.Heat a pan with oil over medium heat, add red chili, urad dal, mustard seeds, hing, curry leaves, stir, and cook for 3 minutes.
3.Add to coconut chutney, stir gently, and serve.

Nutrition: Calories: 114, Fat: 6, Fiber: 5.1, Carbohydrates: 13.9, Protein: 3.4

Coleslaw

Prep Time: 10 minutes **Cook Time:** 0 minutes
Servings: 4

Ingredients:
1 small green cabbage head, shredded
Salt and ground black pepper, to taste
6 tablespoons mayonnaise
1 pinch fennel seed
Juice of ½ lemon
1 tablespoon Dijon mustard

Directions:
1.In a bowl, mix cabbage with salt and lemon juice, stir well, and set aside for 10 minutes.
2.Add salt, pepper, fennel seed, mayonnaise, and mustard to the cabbage. Toss to coat and serve.

Nutrition: Calories: 134, Fat: 7.7, Fiber: 4.6, Carbohydrates: 15.9, Protein: 2.7

Easy Tamarind Chutney

Prep Time: 10 minutes **Cook Time:** 35 minutes
Servings: 10

Ingredients:
1 teaspoon cumin seeds
1 tablespoon canola oil
½ teaspoon garam masala
½ teaspoon asafetida powder
1 teaspoon ground ginger
½ teaspoon fennel seeds
½ teaspoon cayenne pepper
5 tablespoons erythritol
2 cups water
3 tablespoons tamarind paste

Directions:
1.Heat a pan with oil over medium heat, add ginger, cumin, cayenne pepper, asafetida powder, fennel seeds, and garam masala, stir, and cook for 2 minutes.
2.Add water, sweetener, tamarind paste, stir, bring to a boil, reduce heat to low, and simmer chutney for 30 minutes.
3.Transfer to a bowl, and let it cool down before serving.

Nutrition: Calories: 20, Fat: 1.5, Fiber: 02., Carbohydrates: 4.3, Protein: 0.2

Caramelized Bell Peppers

Prep Time: 10 minutes **Cook Time:** 32 minutes
Servings: 4

Ingredients:
1 tablespoon olive oil
1 teaspoon butter
2 red bell peppers, cut into thin strips
2 onions, cut into thin strips
Salt and ground black pepper, to taste
1 teaspoon dried basil

Directions:
1.Heat a pan with butter and oil over medium heat, add onion and bell peppers, stir, and cook for 2 minutes.
2.Reduce temperature and cook for 30 minutes, stirring often.
3.Add the salt, pepper, and basil, stir again, take off heat, and serve.

Nutrition: Calories: 79, Fat: 4.7, Fiber: 2, Carbohydrates: 9.6, Protein: 1.2

Summer Kale

Prep Time: 10 minutes **Cook Time:** 45 minutes
Servings: 4

Ingredients:
2 cups water
1 tablespoon balsamic vinegar
⅓ cup almonds, toasted
3 garlic cloves, peeled and minced
1 bunch kale, steamed, and chopped
1 onion, peeled and chopped
2 tablespoons olive oil

Directions:
1.Heat a pan with oil over medium heat, add onion, stir, and cook for 10 minutes. Add garlic, stir, and cook for 1 minute.
2.Add water and kale, cover pan, and cook for 30 minutes. Add salt, pepper, balsamic vinegar, almonds, toss to coat, divide on plates, and serve.

Nutrition: Calories: 124, Fat: 11, Fiber: 1.7, Carbohydrates: 5.6, Protein: 2.3

Fried Cabbage

Prep Time: 10 minutes **Cook Time:** 15 minutes
Servings: 4

Ingredients:
1½ pound green cabbage, shredded
Salt and ground black pepper, to taste
3. 5 ounces butter
A pinch of sweet paprika

Directions:
1.Heat a pan with butter over medium heat. Add cabbage and cook for 15 minutes, stirring often.
2.Add salt, pepper, paprika, stir, cook for 1 minute, divide on plates, and serve.

Nutrition: Calories: 805, Fat: 86.4, Fiber: 4.3, Carbohydrates: 9.9, Protein: 3.1

Caramelized Red Chard

Prep Time: 10 minutes **Cook Time:** 20 minutes
Servings: 4

Ingredients:
2 tablespoons olive oil
1 onion, peeled and chopped
2 tablespoons capers
Juice of 1 lemon
Salt and ground black pepper, to taste
1 teaspoon erythritol
1 bunch red chard, chopped
¼ cup Kalamata olives, pitted and chopped

Directions:
1.Heat a pan with oil over medium heat, add onions, stir, and brown for 4 minutes.
2.Add erythritol, and stir well. Add olives and chard, stir, and cook for 10 minutes.
3.Add capers, lemon juice, salt, and pepper, stir, and cook for 3 minutes. Divide on plates and serve.

Nutrition: Calories: 83, Fat: 8, Fiber: 1.1, Carbohydrates: 4.8, Protein: 0.6

Lunch Salad

Prep Time: 10 minutes **Cook Time:** 0 minutes
Servings: 2

Ingredients:
1 avocado, pitted, peeled, and sliced
Salt and ground black pepper, to taste
1 tbsp Dijon mustard
2 tbsp keto mayonnaise
1 cup bacon, cooked and crumbled
1 chicken breast, grilled and shredded

Directions:
1.In a salad bowl, mix avocado with bacon and chicken breast, and stir.
2.Add dressing, salt, and pepper, toss to coat, divide into 2 bowls, and serve.

Nutrition: Calories: 334, Fat: 23, Fiber: 4, Carbohydrates: 3, Protein: 18

Green Beans and Avocado

Prep Time: 10 minutes **Cook Time:** 5 minutes
Servings: 4

Ingredients:
⅔ pound green beans, trimmed
Salt and ground black pepper, to taste
3 tablespoons olive oil
2 avocados, pitted and peeled
5 scallions, chopped
½ cup fresh cilantro, chopped

Directions:
1.Heat a pan with oil over medium heat, add green beans, stir, and cook for 4 minutes.
2.Add the salt and pepper, stir, take off heat, and transfer to a bowl.
3.In another bowl, mix avocados with salt and pepper, and mash with a fork.
4.Add onions and stir well. Add this over green beans, toss to coat, and serve.

Nutrition: Calories: 325, Fat: 30.2, Fiber: 9.9, Carbohydrates: 15.5, Protein: 3.7

Creamy Spaghetti Pasta

Prep Time: 10 minutes **Cook Time:** 40 minutes
Servings: 4

Ingredients:
1 spaghetti squash
Salt and ground black pepper, to taste
2 tablespoons butter
1 teaspoon Cajun seasoning
A pinch of cayenne pepper
2 cups heavy cream

Directions:
1.Prick squash with a fork, place on a lined baking sheet and put in an oven at 350°Fand bake for 15 minutes.
2.Take squash out of the oven, set aside to cool, and scoop out the squash flesh.
3.Heat a pan with butter over medium heat, add spaghetti squash, stir, and cook for a couple of minutes.
4.Add salt, pepper, cayenne pepper, Cajun seasoning, stir, and cook for 1 minute.
5.Add heavy cream, stir, cook for 10 minutes, divide on plates, and serve.

Nutrition: Calories: 289, Fat: 28.5, Fiber: 0, Carbohydrates: 8.7, Protein: 1.9

Roasted Olives

Prep Time: 10 minutes **Cook Time:** 20 minutes
Servings: 6

Ingredients:
1 cup black olives, pitted
1 cup Kalamata olives, pitted
1 cup green olives, stuffed with almonds and garlic
¼ cup olive oil
10 garlic cloves
1 tablespoon herbes de Provence
1 teaspoon lemon zest, grated
Ground black pepper, to taste
Fresh thyme, chopped, for serving

Directions:
1.Place black olives, Kalamata olives, and green olives on a lined baking sheet, drizzle oil, garlic, and herbes de Provence, toss to coat, place in an oven at 425°F, and bake for 10 minutes.
2.Stir olives and bake for 10 minutes.
3.Divide olives on plates, sprinkle lemon zest, black pepper, and thyme on top, toss to coat, and serve warm.

Nutrition: Calories: 189, Fat: 18.3, Fiber: 2.5, Carbohydrates: 6.4, Protein: 0.5

Lunch Pizza

Prep Time: 10 minutes **Cook Time:** 7 minutes
Servings: 4

Ingredients:
1 tablespoon olive oil
2 tablespoons butter
2 cups mozzarella cheese, shredded
¼ cup mascarpone cheese
1 tablespoon heavy cream
1 teaspoon garlic, minced
Salt and ground black pepper, to taste
A pinch of lemon pepper
⅓ cup broccoli florets, steamed
Some Asiago cheese, shaved, for serving

Directions:
1.Heat a pan with the oil over medium heat, add pizza cheese mixture, and spread into a circle.
2.Add mozzarella cheese, and spread it into a circle.
3.Cook everything for 5 minutes, and transfer to a plate.
4.Heat the pan with butter over medium heat, add the mascarpone cheese, cream, salt, pepper, lemon pepper, and garlic, stir, and cook for 5 minutes.
5.Drizzle half of the mixture over cheese crust. Add broccoli florets to the pan with rest of the mascarpone mixture, stir, and cook for 1 minute.
6.Add this on top of the pizza, sprinkle with Asiago cheese, and serve.

Nutrition: Calories: 1088, Fat: 81.3, Fiber: 7, Carbohydrates: 10.7, Protein: 76.3

Cheese Dough Pizza

Prep Time: 10 minutes **Cook Time:** 15 minutes
Servings: 2

Ingredients:
1½ cups cheddar cheese, shredded
1½ cups cheese blend
2 beef hot dogs, diced
A drizzle of olive oil
1 pound ground beef
Salt and ground black pepper, to taste
¼ teaspoon paprika
¼ teaspoon Old Bay Seasoning
¼ teaspoon onion powder
¼ teaspoon garlic powder
1 cup lettuce leaves, chopped
1 tablespoon keto mayonnaise
2 tablespoons dill pickles, chopped
2 tablespoons onion, peeled and chopped
½ cup American cheese, shredded
Some mustard, for serving

Directions:
1.Heat a pan with a drizzle of oil over medium heat, add half of the cheese blend, spread into a circle, and top with half of the cheddar cheese.
2.Cook for 5 minutes, transfer to a cutting board, and set aside for a few minutes to cool.
3.Heat the pan again, add the rest of the cheese blend, and spread into a circle.
4.Add the rest of the cheddar, also spread in a circle, cook for 5 minutes, and transfer to a cutting board.
5.Spread mayonnaise over the 2 pizza crusts.
6.Heat the same pan again over medium heat, add the beef, stir, and brown all over.
7.Add salt, pepper, Old Bay Seasoning, paprika, onion powder, and garlic powder, stir, and cook for a few minutes.
8.Add hot dog pieces, stir, and cook for 5 minutes. Spread the lettuce, pickles, American cheese, and onions on the 2 pizza crusts.
9.Divide the beef and hot dog mixture, drizzle with mustard at the end, and serve.

Nutrition: Calories: 1631, Fat: 117.5, Fiber: 0.5, Carbohydrates: 8.4, Protein: 132.5

Vegetable Noodles

Prep Time: 10 minutes **Cook Time:** 20 minutes
Servings: 6

Ingredients:
1 ½ zucchinis, cut with a spiralizer
1 summer squash, cut with a spiralizer
4 oz butternut squash, cut with a spiralizer
4 ounces onion, chopped
6 ounces yellow, orange, and red bell peppers, seeded and cut into thin strips
Salt and ground black pepper, to taste
4 tablespoons bacon fat
3 garlic cloves, peeled and minced

Directions:
1.Spread the zucchini noodles on a lined baking sheet. Add squashes, onion, and bell peppers. Add salt, pepper, garlic and toss to coat.
2.Add bacon fat, toss again, place in an oven at 400ºF, and bake for 20 minutes. Transfer to plates and serve.

Nutrition: Calories: 179, Fat: 8.6, Fiber: 3.6, Carbohydrates: 17.9, Protein: 10

Mustard and Garlic Brussels Sprouts

Prep Time: 10 minutes **Cook Time:** 40 minutes
Servings: 4

Ingredients:
1 pound Brussels sprouts, trimmed, and halved
Salt and ground black pepper, to taste
1 tablespoon coconut aminos
1 tablespoon Dijon mustard
1 tablespoon garlic cloves, peeled and minced
1 tablespoons butter
1 garlic bulb, cloves peeled, and separated
1 tablespoon caraway seeds

Directions:
1.Put the Brussels sprouts on a lined baking sheet. Add minced garlic, whole garlic, butter, mustard, salt, pepper, coconut aminos, and caraway seeds.
2.Toss to coat well, place in an oven at 400ºF, and bake for 40 minutes. Transfer to plates and serve.

Nutrition: Calories: 87, Fat: 3.7, Fiber: 5.1, Carbohydrates: 12.3, Protein: 4.5

Cheese Sauce

Prep Time: 10 minutes **Cook Time:** 12 minutes
Servings: 8

Ingredients:
2 tablespoons butter
¼ cup cream cheese, softened
¼ cup whipping cream
¼ cup cheddar cheese, grated
2 tablespoons water
A pinch of salt
¼ teaspoon cayenne pepper
½ teaspoon sweet paprika
½ teaspoon onion powder
½ teaspoon garlic powder
4 tablespoons fresh parsley, chopped

Directions:
1.Heat a pan with butter over medium heat. Add whipping cream and stir well. Add cream cheese, stir, and bring to a simmer.
2.Take off heat, add cheddar cheese, stir, return to heat, and cook for 3–4 minutes.
3.Add water, a pinch of salt, cayenne pepper, onion powder, garlic powder, paprika, and parsley, stir well, take off heat, and serve.

Nutrition: Calories: 77, Fat: 7.8, Fiber: 0.1, Carbohydrates: 0.5, Protein: 1.6

Sautéed Kohlrabi

Prep Time: 10 minutes **Cook Time:** 10 minutes
Servings: 4

Ingredients:
2 kohlrabi, trimmed and sliced thin
Salt and ground black pepper, to taste
1 tablespoon fresh parsley, chopped
1 tablespoon butter
2 garlic cloves, peeled and minced

Directions:
1.Put kohlrabi in a saucepan with enough water to cover and bring to a boil over medium heat. Cook for 5 minutes, drain, and transfer to a bowl.
2.Heat a pan with the butter over medium heat. Add the garlic, stir, and cook for 1 minute.
3.Add kohlrabi slices, salt, and pepper, and cook until golden brown on both sides.
4.Add parsley, toss to coat, transfer to plates, and serve warm.

Nutrition: Calories: 55, Fat: 3, Fiber: 3.7, Carbohydrates: 6.8, Protein: 1.9

Pizza Rolls

Prep Time: 10 minutes **Cook Time:** 30 minutes
Servings: 6

Ingredients:
¼ cup mixed red and green bell peppers, seeded and chopped
2 cups mozzarella cheese, shredded
1 teaspoon pizza seasoning
2 tablespoons onion, peeled and chopped
1 tomato, cored and chopped
Salt and ground black pepper, to taste
¼ cup tomato paste
½ cup sausage, crumbled and cooked

Directions:
1.Spread mozzarella cheese on a lined and lightly greased baking sheet, sprinkle pizza seasoning on top, place in an oven at 400ºF, and bake for 20 minutes.
2.Take pizza crust out of the oven, spread the sausage, onion, bell peppers, and tomatoes all over, and drizzle tomato paste on top. Place in oven again, and bake for 10 minutes.
3.Take pizza out of the oven, set aside for a couple of minutes, slice into 6 pieces, roll each piece, and serve.

Nutrition: Calories: 99, Fat: 6.7, Fiber: 0.8, Carbohydrates: 3.4, Protein: 6.7

Turnip Fries

Prep Time: 10 minutes **Cook Time:** 25 minutes
Servings: 4

Ingredients:
2 pounds turnips, peeled and cut into sticks
Salt, to taste
¼ cup olive oil
For the seasoning mix:
2 tablespoons chili powder
1 teaspoon garlic powder
½ teaspoon dried oregano
1½ teaspoons onion powder
1½ tablespoons cumin

Directions:
1.In a bowl, mix chili powder with onion powder, garlic powder, cumin, oregano, and stir well. Add parsnips sticks, rub well, and spread on a lined baking sheet.
2.Season with salt, drizzle the oil, toss to coat well, and bake in the oven at 350ºF for 25 minutes.
3.Let parsnip fries cool before serving.

Nutrition: Calories: 230, Fat: 15.1, Fiber: 6.2, Carbohydrates: 23.9, Protein: 4.3

Creamy Cauliflower and Spinach

Prep Time: 10 minutes **Cook Time:** 15 minutes
Servings: 6

Ingredients:
1 cup spinach leaves
3 cups cauliflower florets
¼ cup cream
4 tablespoons butter
Salt and ground black pepper, to taste
½ cup sour cream
1 avocado, pitted and peeled

Directions:
1.In a heatproof bowl, mix spinach with cauliflower florets, place in a microwave, and cook for 15 minutes.
2.Mash avocado with a fork and add to spinach mixture.
3.Add salt, pepper, cream, butter, and sour cream, and blend using an immersion blender.
4.Transfer to plates and serve.

Nutrition: Calories: 197, Fat: 18.9, Fiber: 3.6, Carbohydrates: 6.9, Protein: 2.5

Lunch Tacos

Prep Time: 10 minutes **Cook Time:** 25 minutes
Servings: 3

Ingredients:
2 cups cheddar cheese, grated
1 small avocado, pitted, peeled, and chopped
1 cup taco meat, cooked
2 teaspoons sriracha sauce
¼ cup tomatoes, cored and chopped
Vegetable oil cooking spray
Salt and ground black pepper, to taste

Directions:
1.Spray cooking oil on lined baking dish. Spread cheddar cheese on the baking sheet, place in an oven at 400ºF, and bake for 15 minutes.
2.Spread taco meat over cheese, and bake for 10 minutes.
3.In a bowl, mix avocado with tomatoes, sriracha sauce, salt, pepper, and stir.
4.Spread over the taco and cheddar layers, let the tacos cool, slice using a pizza cutter, and serve.

Nutrition: Calories: 400, Fat: 23, Fiber: 0, Carbohydrates: 2, Protein: 37

Taco Salad

Prep Time: 10 minutes **Cook Time:** 20 minutes
Servings: 4

Ingredients:
¼ cup fresh cilantro, chopped
2 avocados, pitted, peeled, and cut into chunks
1 tablespoon lime juice
¼ cup white onion, peeled and chopped
1 teaspoon garlic, minced
Salt and ground black pepper, to taste
6 cherry tomatoes, cut in quarters
½ cup water
2–pound ground beef
2 cups sour cream
¼ cup taco seasoning
2 cups lettuce leaves, shredded
1 tsp cayenne pepper powder
2 cups cheddar cheese, shredded

Directions:
1.In a bowl, mix cilantro with lime juice, avocado, onion, tomatoes, salt, pepper, and garlic, stir well, and set aside in the refrigerator.
2.Heat a pan over medium heat, add beef, stir, and brown for 10 minutes.
3.Add taco seasoning and water, stir, and cook over medium–low heat for 10 minutes.
4.Divide mixture into 4 serving bowls.
5.Add sour cream, avocado mixture, lettuce pieces, and cheddar cheese.
6.Drizzle with cayenne pepper at the end and serve.

Nutrition: Calories: 1141, Fat: 77, Fiber: 9.3, Carbohydrates: 23.3, Protein: 90.3

Stuffed Peppers

Prep Time: 10 minutes **Cook Time:** 40 minutes
Servings: 4

Ingredients:
4 big banana peppers, peeled, tops cut off, and cut into half lengthwise
1 tablespoon butter
Salt and ground black pepper, to taste
½ teaspoon herbs de Provence
1 pound sweet sausage, chopped
3 tablespoons onions, peeled and chopped
Tomato puree, to serve
A drizzle of olive oil

Directions:
1.Season banana peppers with salt and pepper, drizzle oil, rub well, and bake in the oven at 350ºF for 20 minutes.
2.Heat a pan over medium heat, add sausage pieces, stir, and cook for 5 minutes.
3.Add onion, herbs de Provence, salt, pepper, butter, stir well, and cook for 5 minutes.
4.Take peppers out of the oven, fill them with sausage mixture, place them in an oven–proof dish, drizzle tomato puree, place in an oven again, and bake for 10 minutes. Serve hot.

Nutrition: Calories: 486, Fat: 39.2, Fiber: 1.8, Carbohydrates: 11.2, Protein: 22,3

Bacon and Zucchini Noodle Salad

Prep Time: 10 minutes **Cook Time:** 0 minutes
Servings: 2

Ingredients:
1 cup baby spinach
4 cups zucchini noodles
⅓ cup blue cheese, crumbled
⅓ cup blue cheese dressing
½ cup bacon, cooked and crumbled
Ground black pepper, to taste

Directions:
1.In a salad bowl, mix spinach with zucchini noodles, bacon, blue cheese, and toss.
2.Add cheese dressing and black pepper to taste, toss well to coat, divide into 2 bowls, and serve.

Nutrition: Calories: 500, Fat: 41.6, Fiber: 3.1, Carbohydrates: 12.9, Protein: 22

Chili Pepper Burger

Prep Time: 10 minutes **Cook Time:** 30 minutes
Servings: 4

Ingredients:
For the sauce:
4 chili peppers, chopped
1 cup water
1 cup almond butter
1 teaspoon swerve
6 tablespoons coconut aminos
4 garlic cloves, peeled and minced
1 tablespoon rice vinegar
For the burgers:
4 pepper jack cheese slices
1½ pounds ground beef
1 onion, peeled and sliced
8 bacon slices
8 lettuce leaves
Salt and ground black pepper, to taste

Directions:
1.Heat a pan with the almond butter over medium heat. Add water, stir well, and bring to a simmer. Add coconut aminos and stir well.
2.In a food processor, mix chili peppers with garlic, swerve, vinegar, and blend well. Add to almond butter mixture, stir well, take off heat, and set aside.
3.In a bowl, mix beef with salt and pepper, stir, and shape into 4 patties. Place in a pan then transfer to a preheated broiler, and broil for 7 minutes.
4.Flip the burgers and broil them for 7 minutes.
5.Place cheese slices on burgers, place under a broiler, and broil for 4 minutes.
6.Heat a pan over medium heat, add bacon slices, and fry them for a couple of minutes.
7.Place 2 lettuce leaves on a dish, add the 1 burger on top, then 1 onion slice and 1 bacon slice, and top with some almond butter sauce.
8.Repeat with the rest of the lettuce leaves, burgers, onion, bacon, and sauce.

Nutrition: Calories: 690, Fat: 37.8, Fiber: 1.3, Carbohydrates: 9.3, Protein: 74.1

Steak Salad

Prep Time: 10 minutes **Cook Time:** 20 minutes
Servings: 4

Ingredients:
1½ pound steak, sliced thin
3 tablespoons avocado oil
Salt and ground black pepper, to taste
¼ cup balsamic vinegar
6 ounces sweet onion, peeled and chopped
1 lettuce head, chopped
2 garlic cloves, peeled and minced
4 ounces mushrooms, sliced
1 avocado, pitted, peeled, and sliced
3 ounces sundried tomatoes, cored and chopped
1 yellow bell pepper, seeded and sliced
1 orange bell pepper, seeded and sliced
1 teaspoon Italian seasoning
1 teaspoon red pepper flakes
1 teaspoon onion powder

Directions:
1.In a bowl, mix steak pieces with some salt, pepper, balsamic vinegar, toss to coat, and set aside.
2.Heat a pan with the avocado oil over medium–low heat, add mushrooms, garlic, salt, pepper, onion, stir, and cook for 20 minutes.
3.In a bowl, mix lettuce leaves with bell peppers, sundried tomatoes, avocado, and stir.
4.Season steak pieces with onion powder, pepper flakes, and Italian seasoning.
5.Place steak pieces in a broiling pan, place under a preheated broiler, and cook for 5 minutes.
6.Divide the steak pieces on plates, add lettuce, and avocado salad on the side, and top everything with onion and mushroom mixture.

Nutrition: Calories: 1516, Fat: 50.1, Fiber: 7.2, Carbohydrates: 25.3, Protein: 231.1

Beef Brisket Burgers

Prep Time: 10 minutes **Cook Time:** 25 minutes
Servings: 8

Ingredients:
1 pound ground beef brisket
1 pound ground beef
Salt and ground black pepper, to taste
½ cup butter
1 tablespoon garlic, minced
1 tablespoon Italian seasoning
2 tablespoons mayonnaise
1 tablespoon butter
2 tablespoons olive oil
1 onion, peeled and chopped
1 tablespoon water

Directions:
1.In a bowl, mix brisket with ground beef, salt, pepper, Italian seasoning, garlic, mayonnaise, and stir well.
2.Shape 8 patties and make a pocket in each. Stuff each burger with a butter slice and seal.
3.Heat a pan with olive oil over medium heat, add onions, stir, and cook for 2 minutes.
4.Add water, stir, and push to one corner of the pan.
5.Place burgers in pan with the onions and cook over medium–low heat for 10 minutes.
6.Flip, add butter, and cook for 10 minutes.
7.Divide burgers on buns and serve them with caramelized onions on top.

Nutrition: Calories: 423, Fat: 25.7, Fiber: 0.3, Carbohydrates: 2.7, Protein: 43.4

Zucchini with Cheese

Prep Time: 10 minutes **Cook Time:** 5 minutes
Servings: 1

Ingredients:
1 tablespoon olive oil
3 tablespoons butter
2 cups zucchini, cut with a spiralizer
1 teaspoon red pepper flakes
1 tablespoon garlic, minced
1 tablespoon red bell pepper, seeded and chopped
Salt and ground black pepper, to taste
1 tablespoon fresh basil, chopped
¼ cup Asiago cheese, shaved
¼ cup Parmesan cheese, grated

Directions:
1.Heat a pan with oil and butter over medium heat, add the garlic, bell pepper, and pepper flakes, stir, and cook for 1 minute.
2.Add zucchini noodles, stir, and cook for 2 minutes.
3.Add basil, Parmesan cheese, salt, pepper, stir, and cook for a few seconds.
4.Take off heat, transfer to a bowl, and serve with Asiago cheese on top.

Nutrition: Calories: 870, Fat: 66, Fiber: 7.2, Carbohydrates: 28.9, Protein: 47.5

Chicken Salad

Prep Time: 10 minutes **Cook Time:** 0 minutes
Servings: 3

Ingredients:
1 green onion, peeled and chopped
1 celery stalk, chopped
1 egg, hard–boiled, peeled and chopped
5 ounces chicken breast, roasted and chopped
2 tablespoons fresh parsley, chopped
½ tablespoons dill relish
Salt and ground black pepper, to taste
⅓ cup mayonnaise
A pinch of garlic powder
1 teaspoon mustard

Directions:
1.In a food processor, mix parsley with onion, celery, and pulse well. Transfer to a bowl and set aside.
2.Put chicken in a food processor, blend well, and add to the bowl with the vegetables. Add egg pieces, salt, pepper, and stir.
3.Add mustard, mayonnaise, dill relish, and garlic powder, toss to coat, and serve.

Nutrition: Calories: 184, Fat: 11.7, Fiber: 0.4, Carbohydrates: 7.3, Protein: 12.5

Fennel and Chicken Salad

Prep Time: 10 minutes **Cook Time:** 0 minutes
Servings: 4

Ingredients:
3 chicken breasts, boneless, skinless, cooked, and chopped
2 tablespoons walnut oil
¼ cup walnuts, toasted and chopped
1½ cup fennel, chopped
2 tablespoons lemon juice
¼ cup mayonnaise
2 tablespoons lamb with fronds, chopped
Salt and ground black pepper, to taste
A pinch of cayenne pepper

Directions:
1.In a bowl, mix fennel with chicken, walnuts, and stir. In another bowl, mix mayo with salt, pepper, fennel fronds, walnut oil, lemon juice, cayenne, garlic, and stir well.
2.Pour over chicken, fennel mixture and toss to coat well, and keep in the refrigerator until ready to serve.

Nutrition: Calories: 624, Fat: 32.7, Fiber: 4.3, Carbohydrates: 13.2, Protein: 65.7

Pesto Chicken Salad

Prep Time: 10 minutes **Cook Time:** 0 minutes
Servings: 4

Ingredients:
1 pound chicken meat, cooked, and cubed
Salt and ground black pepper, to taste
10 cherry tomatoes, halved
6 bacon slices, cooked and crumbled
¼ cup mayonnaise
1 avocado, pitted, peeled, and cubed
1 garlic clove, peeled and minced
2 tablespoons pesto

Directions:
1.In a salad bowl, mix chicken with bacon, avocado, tomatoes, salt, and pepper, and stir.
2.Add mayonnaise and garlic pesto, toss well to coat, and serve.

Nutrition: Calories: 177, Fat: 11.1, Fiber: 2.1, Carbohydrates: 6, Protein: 13.7

Steak Spicy Salad

Prep Time: 10 minutes **Cook Time:** 10 minutes
Servings: 1

Ingredients:
4 ounces beef steak
2 cups lettuce leaves, shredded
Salt and ground black pepper, to taste
Vegetable oil cooking spray
2 tablespoons fresh cilantro, chopped
2 radishes, sliced
⅓ cup red cabbage, shredded
For the salad dressing:
3 garlic cloves, peeled and minced
½ teaspoon Worcestershire sauce
1 tablespoon mustard
½ cup apple cider vinegar
¼ cup water
½ cup olive oil
¼ teaspoon hot sauce
Salt and ground black pepper, to taste

Directions:
1.In a bowl, mix garlic cloves with Worcestershire sauce, mustard, cider vinegar, water, olive oil, salt, pepper, and hot sauce, whisk, and set aside.
2.Heat a broiler over medium–high heat, spray cooking oil, add steak, season with salt, pepper, cook for 4 minutes, flip, cook for 4 minutes, take off heat, set aside to cool down, and cut into thin strips.
3.In a salad bowl, mix lettuce with cilantro, cabbage, radishes, and steak strips. Add 1 tablespoon of olive oil, toss to coat, and serve.

Nutrition: Calories: 1191, Fat: 111.4, Fiber: 3.3, Carbohydrates: 13.5, Protein: 38.7

Easy Stuffed Avocado

Prep Time: 10 minutes **Cook Time:** 0 minutes
Servings: 1

Ingredients:
1 avocado
4 ounces canned sardines, drained
1 green onion, peeled and chopped
1 tablespoon mayonnaise
1 tablespoon lemon juice
Salt and ground black pepper, to taste
¼ teaspoon turmeric

Directions:
1.Cut avocado in half, scoop out the flesh and put in a bowl.
2.Mix with the sardines and mash with a fork.
3.Mix with onion, lemon juice, turmeric, salt, pepper, and mayonnaise.
4.Stir everything, divide into avocado halves, and serve.

Nutrition: Calories: 712, Fat: 57.2, Fiber: 13.8, Carbohydrates: 22.2, Protein: 32.3

Easy Crab Cakes

Prep Time: 10 minutes **Cook Time:** 12 minutes
Servings: 6

Ingredients:
1 pound crabmeat
¼ cup fresh parsley, chopped
Salt and ground black pepper, to taste
2 green onions, chopped
¼ cup fresh cilantro, chopped
1 teaspoon jalapeño pepper, minced
1 teaspoon lemon juice
1 teaspoon Worcestershire sauce
1 teaspoon Old Bay Seasoning
½ teaspoon dry mustard
½ cup mayonnaise
1 egg
2 tablespoons olive oil

Directions:
1.In a large bowl, mix crab meat with salt, pepper, parsley, green onions, cilantro, jalapeño, lemon juice, Old Bay seasoning, dry mustard, Worcestershire sauce, and stir well.
2.In another bowl, mix egg with mayonnaise and whisk. Add to the crabmeat mixture and stir.
3.Shape 6 patties from this mixture, and place them on a plate.
4.Heat a pan with the oil over medium–high heat, add 3 of the crab cakes, cook for 3 minutes, flip, cook them for 3 minutes, and transfer to paper towels.
5.Repeat with the other 3 crab cakes, drain the excess grease, and serve.

Nutrition: Calories: 204, Fat: 12.4, Fiber: 0.7, Carbohydrates: 16.9, Protein: 7.1

Lunch Muffins

Prep Time: 10 minutes **Cook Time:** 45 minutes
Servings: 13

Ingredients:
6 egg yolks
2 tablespoons coconut aminos
½ pound mushrooms
¾ cup coconut flour
1 pound ground beef
Salt, to taste

Directions:
1.In a food processor, mix mushrooms with salt, coconut aminos, egg yolks, and blend well.
2.In a bowl, mix beef meat with some salt and stir.
3.Add mushroom mixture to beef and stir. Add coconut flour and stir again. Divide into 13 cupcake cups, place in an oven at 350ºF, and bake for 45 minutes. Serve warm.

Nutrition: Calories: 98, Fat: 4.4, Fiber: 0.5, Carbohydrates: 1.6, Protein: 12.5

Pork Pie

Prep Time: 10 minutes **Cook Time:** 50 minutes
Servings: 6

Ingredients:
For the pie crust:
2 cups pork crackling
¼ cup flax meal
1 cup almond flour
2 eggs
A pinch of salt
For the filling:
1 cup cheddar cheese, grated
4 eggs
12 ounces pork loin, chopped
6 bacon slices
½ cup cream cheese
1 onion, peeled and chopped
¼ cup fresh chives, chopped
2 garlic cloves, peeled and minced
Salt and ground black pepper, to taste
2 tablespoons butter

Directions:
1.In a food processor, mix the crackling with almond flour, flax meal, 2 eggs, salt, and blend until you obtain a dough.
2.Transfer to a pie pan, and press on the bottom firmly. Place in an oven at 350ºF, and bake for 15 minutes.
3.Heat a pan with butter over medium–high heat, add garlic and onion, stir, and cook for 5 minutes. Add bacon, stir, and cook for 5 minutes.
4.Add pork loin, cook until brown on all sides, and take off heat. In a bowl, mix eggs with salt, pepper, cheddar cheese, cream cheese, and blend well.
5.Add chives and stir again.
6.Spread pork into pie pan, add the eggs mixture, place in an oven at 350ºF, and bake for 25 minutes.
7.Let the pie cool down for a couple of minutes and serve.

Nutrition: Calories: 785, Fat: 60, Fiber: 3.4, Carbohydrates: 7.5, Protein: 55.6

Lunch Curry

Prep Time: 10 minutes **Cook Time:** 1 hour
Servings: 4

Ingredients:
3 tomatoes, cored and chopped
2 tablespoons olive oil
1 cup chicken stock
14 ounces canned coconut milk
1 tablespoon lime juice
Salt and ground black pepper, to taste
2 pounds chicken thighs, boneless, skinless, and cubed
2 garlic cloves, peeled and minced
1 cup onion, peeled and chopped
3 red chilies, chopped
1 ounce peanuts, toasted
1 tablespoon water
1 tablespoon fresh ginger, grated
2 teaspoons coriander
1 teaspoon ground cinnamon
1 teaspoon turmeric
1 teaspoon cumin
½ teaspoon ground black pepper
1 teaspoon ground fennel seeds

Directions:
1.In a food processor, mix onion with garlic, peanuts, red chilies, water, ginger, coriander, cinnamon, turmeric, cumin, fennel, and black pepper. Blend until you obtain a paste and set aside.
2.Heat a pan with olive oil over medium–high heat, add the spice paste you've made, stir well, and heat for a few seconds.
3.Add chicken pieces, stir, and cook for 2 minutes.
4.Add stock, tomatoes, stir, reduce heat to low, and cook for 30 minutes.
5.Add coconut milk, stir, and cook for 20 minutes.
6.Add salt, pepper, lime juice, stir, divide into bowls, and serve.

Nutrition: Calories: 804, Fat: 51.6, Fiber: 5.4, Carbohydrates: 16.1, Protein: 71.5

Lunch Pâte

Prep Time: 10 minutes **Cook Time:** 0 minutes
Servings: 1

Ingredients:
4 ounces chicken livers, sautéed
½ teaspoon fresh thyme, chopped
½ teaspoon fresh sage, chopped
½ teaspoon fresh oregano, chopped
Salt and ground black pepper, to taste
3 tablespoons butter
3 radishes, sliced thin

Directions:
1.In a food processor, mix chicken livers with the thyme, sage, oregano, butter, salt, and pepper, and blend well.
2.Top with radishes slices and serve.

Nutrition: Calories: 497, Fat: 41.9, Fiber: 0.2, Carbohydrates: 1.5, Protein: 28.2

Chicken Chowder

Prep Time: 10 minutes **Cook Time:** 4 hours
Servings: 4

Ingredients:
1 pound chicken thighs, skinless and boneless
10 ounces canned diced tomatoes
1 cup chicken stock
8 ounces cream cheese
Juice from 1 lime
Salt and ground black pepper, to taste
1 jalapeño pepper, chopped
1 onion, peeled and chopped
2 tablespoons fresh cilantro, chopped
1 garlic clove, peeled and minced
Cheddar cheese, shredded, for serving
Lime wedges, for serving

Directions:
1.In a slow cooker, mix chicken with the tomatoes, stock, cream cheese, salt, pepper, lime juice, jalapeño, onion, garlic, cilantro, stir, cover, and cook on high for 4 hours.
2.Uncover slow cooker, shred the meat, divide into bowls, and serve with cheddar cheese on top and lime wedges on the side.

Nutrition: Calories: 447, Fat: 28.5, Fiber: 2.1, Carbohydrates: 9.3, Protein: 38.5

Coconut Soup

Prep Time: 10 minutes **Cook Time:** 30 minutes
Servings: 2

Ingredients:
4 cups chicken stock
3 lime leaves
1½ cups coconut milk
1 teaspoon fried lemongrass
1 cup fresh cilantro, chopped
1–inchfresh ginger, peeled and grated
4 Thai chilies, dried and chopped
Salt and ground black pepper, to taste
4 ounces shrimp, peeled and deveined
2 tablespoons onion, chopped
1 tablespoon coconut oil
2 tablespoons mushrooms, chopped
1 tablespoon fish sauce
1 tablespoon fresh cilantro, chopped
Juice from 1 lime

Directions:
1.In a pot, mix chicken stock with coconut milk, lime leaves, lemongrass, Thai chilies, 1 cup cilantro, ginger, salt, pepper, stir, bring to a simmer over medium heat, cook for 20 minutes, strain, and return to pot.
2.Heat up soup again over medium heat, add coconut oil, shrimp, fish sauce, mushrooms, onions, stir, and cook for 10 minutes.
3.Add lime juice and 1 tablespoon cilantro, stir, ladle into bowls, and serve.

Nutrition: Calories: 1673, Fat: 166.3, Fiber: 15, Carbohydrates: 40.6, Protein: 30.3

Sausage Stuffing

Prep Time: 10 minutes **Cook Time:** 4 hours and 20 minutes
Servings: 8

Ingredients:
2 cups almond flour
2 tablespoons whey protein powder
¼ cup coconut flour
½ teaspoon garlic powder
2 teaspoons baking powder
1¼ cups cheddar cheese, shredded
2 eggs
¼ cup melted butter
¾ cup water
For the stuffing:
½ cup onion, peeled and chopped
2 tablespoons butter
1 red bell pepper, seeded and chopped
1 jalapeño pepper, chopped
Salt and ground black pepper, to taste
12 ounces sausage, chopped
2 eggs
¾ cup chicken stock
¼ cup whipping cream

Directions:
1.In a bowl, mix coconut flour with whey protein, almond flour, garlic powder, baking powder, 1 cup cheddar cheese, and stir.
2.Add water, 2 eggs, ¼ cup butter, stir well. Transfer to a greased baking pan, sprinkle rest of the cheddar cheese, place in an oven at 325ºF, and bake for 30 minutes.
3.Let bread cool down for 15 minutes, and cube it.
4.Spread bread cubes on a lined baking sheet, place in an oven at 200ºF, and bake for 3 hours.
5.Take bread cubes out of the oven and set aside.
6.Heat a pan with 2 tablespoons butter over medium heat, add onion, stir, and cook for 4 minutes.
7.Add jalapeño and red bell pepper, stir, and cook for 5 minutes.
8.Add salt and pepper, stir, and transfer everything to a bowl.
9.Heat the same pan over medium heat, add sausage, stir, and cook for 10 minutes.
10.Transfer sausage to the bowl with the vegetables, stock, bread, and stir. In a separate bowl, whisk 2 eggs with some salt, pepper, and whipping cream.
11.Add this to the sausage and bread mixture, stir, transfer to a greased baking pan, place in an oven at 325ºF, and bake for 30 minutes. Serve hot.

Nutrition: Calories: 505, Fat: 43.6, Fiber: 1.3, Carbohydrates: 5.4, Protein: 24.2

Zucchini Noodle Soup

Prep Time: 10 minutes **Cook Time:** 15 minutes
Servings: 8

Ingredients:
1 onion, peeled and chopped
2 garlic cloves, peeled and minced
1 jalapeño pepper, chopped
1 tablespoon coconut oil
1½ tablespoons curry paste
6 cups chicken stock
15 ounces canned coconut milk
1 pound chicken breasts, boneless, skinless, and sliced
1 red bell pepper, seeded and sliced
2 tablespoons fish sauce
2 zucchini, cut with a spiralizer
½ cup fresh cilantro, chopped
Lime wedges, for serving

Directions:
1.Heat a pot with oil over medium heat, add onion, stir, and cook for 5 minutes.
2.Add garlic, jalapeño, and curry paste, stir, and cook for 1 minute.
3.Add stock, coconut milk, stir, and bring to a boil.
4.Add red bell pepper, chicken, fish sauce, stir, and simmer for 4 minutes.
5.Add cilantro, stir, cook for 1 minute, and take off the heat.
6.Divide zucchini noodles into soup bowls, add the soup on top, and serve with lime wedges on the side.

Nutrition: Calories: 343, Fat: 25.2, Fiber: 2.3, Carbohydrates: 11, Protein: 19.9

Spinach Rolls

Prep Time: 20 minutes **Cook Time:** 15 minutes
Servings: 16

Ingredients:
6 tablespoons coconut flour
½ cup almond flour
2, and ½ cups mozzarella cheese, shredded
2 eggs
A pinch of salt
For the filling:
4 ounces cream cheese
6 ounces spinach, torn
A drizzle of avocado oil
A pinch of salt
¼ cup Parmesan cheese, grated
Mayonnaise, for serving

Directions:
1.Heat a pan with oil over medium heat, add spinach, and cook for 2 minutes. Add Parmesan cheese, a pinch of salt, cream cheese, stir well, take off the heat, and set aside.
2.Put mozzarella cheese in a heatproof bowl and microwave for 30 seconds. Add eggs, salt, coconut, almond flour, and stir.
3.Place dough on a lined cutting board, place parchment paper on top, and flatten dough with a rolling pin.
4.Divide dough into 16 rectangles, spread spinach mixture on each, and roll them into cigar shapes.
5.Place all rolls on a lined baking sheet, place in oven at 350ºF, and bake for 15 minutes.
6.Let rolls cool down for a few minutes before serving them with some mayonnaise on top.

Nutrition: Calories: 113, Fat: 7.3, Fiber: 2.6, Carbohydrates: 5.1, Protein: 7.3

Sausage Gravy

Prep Time: 10 minutes **Cook Time:** 10 minutes
Servings: 4

Ingredients:
4 ounces sausages, chopped
Salt and ground black pepper, to taste
1 cup heavy cream
2 tablespoons butter
½ teaspoon guar gum

Directions:
1.Heat a pan over medium heat, add sausage pieces, stir, cook for 4 minutes, transfer to a plate.
2.Return pan to the heat, add butter, and melt it.
3.Add cream, salt, pepper, guar gum, stir and cook until it begins to thicken.
4.Return sausage to pan, stir well, take off heat, and serve.

Nutrition: Calories: 251, Fat: 24.9, Fiber: 0, Carbohydrates: 0.8, Protein: 6.2

Steak Bowl

Prep Time: 15 minutes **Cook Time:** 8 minutes
Servings: 4

Ingredients:
16 ounces skirt steak
4 ounces pepper jack cheese, shredded
1 cup sour cream
Salt and ground black pepper, to taste
½ cup fresh cilantro, chopped
1 tbsp tomato paste
1 tbsp cider vinegar
1 tsp chipotle powder
For the guacamole:
¼ cup onion, chopped
2 avocados, pitted and peeled
Juice from 1 lime
1 tablespoon olive oil
6 cherry tomatoes, cored and chopped
1 garlic clove, peeled and minced
1 tablespoon fresh cilantro, chopped
Salt and ground black pepper, to taste

Directions:
1.Put avocados in a bowl and mash with a fork. Add tomatoes, onion, garlic, salt, pepper, and stir well.
2.Add olive oil, lime juice, and 1 tablespoon cilantro, stir again well, and set aside.
3.Heat a pan over high heat, add steak, season with salt, pepper, cook for 4 minutes on each side, transfer to a cutting board, set aside to cool, and cut into thin strips.
4.In a bowl, mix tomato paste, cider vinegar, and chipotle powder to make chipotle adobo sauce.
5.Divide steak into 4 bowls, add cheese, sour cream, and guacamole on top, and serve with a splash of chipotle adobo sauce.

Nutrition: Calories: 743, Fat: 56.1, Fiber: 9.3, Carbohydrates: 20, Protein: 43

Mushroom and Hemp Pilaf

Prep Time: 10 minutes **Cook Time:** 20 minutes
Servings: 4

Ingredients:
2 tablespoons butter
¼ cup almonds, sliced
3 mushrooms, chopped
1 cup hemp seeds
Salt and ground black pepper, to taste
½ teaspoon garlic powder
½ cup chicken stock
¼ teaspoon dried parsley

Directions:
1.Heat a pan with the butter over medium heat, add almonds and mushrooms, stir, and cook for 4 minutes.
2.Add hemp seeds and stir. Add salt, pepper, parsley, garlic powder, stock, stir, reduce the heat, cover the pan, and simmer until stock is absorbed.
3.Divide on plates and serve.

Nutrition: Calories: 196, Fat: 17.4, Fiber: 1.5, Carbohydrates: 3.3, Protein: 8.2

Meatball Pilaf

Prep Time: 10 minutes **Cook Time:** 30 minutes
Servings: 4

Ingredients:
12 ounces cauliflower florets
Salt and ground black pepper, to taste
1 egg
1 pound ground lamb
1 teaspoon fennel seed
1 teaspoon paprika
1 teaspoon garlic powder
1 onion, peeled and chopped
2 garlic cloves, peeled and minced
2 tablespoons coconut oil
1 bunch fresh mint, chopped
1 tablespoon lemon zest
4 ounces goats cheese, crumbled

Directions:
1.Put the cauliflower florets in a food processor, add salt and pulse well.
2.Grease a pan with some coconut oil, heat over medium heat, add cauliflower rice, cook for 8 minutes, season with some salt and pepper, take off the heat and keep warm.
3.In a bowl, mix the lamb with salt, pepper, egg, paprika, garlic powder, fennel seed, and stir well. Shape 12 meatballs and place them on a plate.
4.Heat a pan with the coconut oil over medium heat, add onion, stir, and cook for 6 minutes. Add garlic, stir, and cook for 1 minute.
5.Add meatballs, cook them well on all sides, and take off the heat.
6.Divide cauliflower rice on plates, add meatballs and onion mixture on top, sprinkle the mint, lemon zest, and goat cheese at the end, and serve.

Nutrition: Calories: 345, Fat: 16.5, Fiber: 3.2, Carbohydrates: 8.7, Protein: 35.6

Broccoli Soup

Prep Time: 10 minutes **Cook Time:** 30 minutes
Servings: 4

Ingredients:
1 white onion, peeled and chopped
1 tablespoon butter
2 cups vegetable stock
Salt and ground black pepper, to taste
2 cups water
2 garlic cloves, peeled and minced
1 cup heavy cream
8 ounces cheddar cheese, grated
12 ounces broccoli florets
½ teaspoon paprika

Directions:
1.Heat a saucepan with butter over medium heat, add onion and garlic, stir, and cook for 5 minutes.
2.Add stock, cream, water, salt, pepper, paprika, stir, and bring to a boil.
3.Add broccoli, stir, and simmer the soup for 25 minutes.
4.Transfer to a food processor and blend well. Add cheese and blend again.
5.Divide into soup bowls and serve hot.

Nutrition: Calories: 400, Fat: 33.1, Fiber: 2.9, Carbohydrates: 10.4, Protein: 17.6

Green Bean Salad

Prep Time: 10 minutes **Cook Time:** 5 minutes
Servings: 8

Ingredients:
2 tablespoons white wine vinegar
1½ tablespoons mustard
Salt and ground black pepper, to taste
2 pounds green beans
⅓ cup extra virgin olive oil
1½ cups fennel, sliced thin
4 ounces goats cheese, crumbled
¾ cup walnuts, toasted and chopped

Directions:
1.Put water in a saucepan, add some salt, and bring to a boil over medium–high heat.
2.Add green beans, cook for 5 minutes, and transfer them to a bowl filled with ice water.
3.Drain green beans well and put them in a salad bowl. Add walnuts, fennel, and goat cheese and toss gently.
4.In a bowl, mix vinegar with mustard, salt, pepper, oil, and whisk. Pour this over the salad, toss to coat well, and serve.

Nutrition: Calories: 244, Fat: 19.1, Fiber: 6.5, Carbohydrates: 14.1, Protein: 8.6

Twice–baked Zucchini

Prep Time: 10 minutes **Cook Time:** 30 minutes
Servings: 4

Ingredients:
2 zucchinis, cut into half and each half in half lengthwise
¼ cup onion, peeled and chopped
½ cup cheddar cheese, shredded
4 bacon strips, cooked and crumbled
¼ cup sour cream
2 ounces cream cheese, softened
1 tablespoon jalapeño pepper, chopped
Salt and ground black pepper, to taste
2 tablespoons butter

Directions:
1.Scoop the zucchinis, place flesh in a bowl, and arrange zucchini cups in a baking dish.
2.Add onion, cheddar cheese, crumbled bacon, jalapeño, salt, pepper, sour cream, cream cheese, and butter to the bowl.
3.Whisk well, fill zucchini quarters with this mixture, place in an oven at 350°F, and bake for 30 minutes.
4.Divide zucchini on plates, and serve.

Nutrition: Calories: 237, Fat: 21.3, Fiber: 1.2, Carbohydrates: 5.1, Protein: 7.6

Pumpkin Soup

Prep Time: 10 minutes **Cook Time:** 20 minutes
Servings: 6

Ingredients:
½ cup onion, peeled and chopped
2 tablespoons olive oil
1 tbsp tomato paste
1 tbsp cider vinegar
1 tsp chipotle powder
1 garlic clove, peeled and minced
1 teaspoon cumin
1 teaspoon coriander
A pinch of allspice
2 cups pumpkin puree
Salt and ground black pepper, to taste
1 quart chicken stock
½ cup heavy cream
2 teaspoons vinegar
2 teaspoons stevia

Directions:
1.Heat a pot with the oil over medium heat, add onions and garlic, stir, and cook for 4 minutes.
2.Add stevia, coriander, tomato paste, vinegar, chipotle powder, and cumin, stir, and cook for 2 minutes.
3.Add stock and pumpkin puree, stir, and cook for 5 minutes.
4.Blend soup well using an immersion blender and then mix with salt, pepper, heavy cream, and vinegar.
5.Stir, cook for 5 minutes, and divide into bowls, and serve.

Nutrition: Calories: 109, Fat: 8.6, Fiber: 2.7, Carbohydrates: 9.1, Protein: 1.4

Green Bean Casserole

Prep Time: 10 minutes **Cook Time:** 35 minutes
Servings: 8

Ingredients:
1 pound green beans, halved
Salt and ground black pepper, to taste
½ cup almond flour
2 tablespoons butter
8 ounces mushrooms, chopped
4 ounces onion, peeled and chopped
2 shallots, peeled and chopped
3 garlic cloves, peeled and minced
½ cup chicken stock
½ cup heavy cream
¼ cup Parmesan cheese, grated
Avocado oil for frying

Directions:
1.Put some water in a saucepan, add salt, bring to a boil over medium–high heat, add green beans, cook for 5 minutes, transfer to a bowl filled with ice water, cool down, drain well, and set aside.
2.In a bowl, mix the shallots with the onions, almond flour, salt, and pepper, and toss to coat.
3.Heat a pan with some avocado oil over medium–high heat, add onions, shallots mixture, fry until golden. Transfer to paper towels, and drain the grease.
4.Heat the pan over medium heat, add butter and melt it. Add garlic and mushrooms, stir, and cook for 5 minutes.
5.Add stock and heavy cream, stir, bring to a boil, and simmer until it thickens. Add Parmesan cheese and green beans, toss to coat, and take off heat.
6.Transfer mixture to a baking dish, sprinkle some crispy onions mixture all over, place in an oven at 400ºF, and bake for 15 minutes. Serve warm.

Nutrition: Calories: 104, Fat: 7.1, Fiber: 2.7, Carbohydrates: 8.6, Protein: 3.5

Baby Mushrooms

Prep Time: 10 minutes **Cook Time:** 30 minutes
Servings: 4

Ingredients:
4 tablespoons butter
16 ounces baby mushrooms
Salt and ground black pepper, to taste
3 tablespoons dried onion flakes
3 tablespoons dried parsley
1 teaspoon garlic powder

Directions:
1.In a bowl, mix parsley flakes with onion, salt, pepper, garlic powder, and stir.
2.In another bowl, mix mushroom with melted butter and toss to coat.
3.Add seasoning mixture, toss well, spread on a lined baking sheet, place in an oven at 300ºF, bake for 30 minutes, and serve.

Nutrition: Calories: 139, Fat: 11.5, Fiber: 0, Carbohydrates: 3.8, Protein: 3.9

Mixed Vegetable Dish

Prep Time: 10 minutes **Cook Time:** 10 minutes
Servings: 4

Ingredients:
14 ounces mushrooms, sliced
3 ounces broccoli florets
6 tablespoons olive oil
Salt and ground black pepper, to taste
3 ounces bell pepper, seeded and cut into strips
3 ounces spinach, torn
2 tablespoons garlic, minced
2 tablespoons pumpkin seeds
A pinch of red pepper flakes

Directions:
1.Heat up a pan with the oil over medium–high heat, add the garlic, stir, and cook for 1 minute.
2.Add the mushrooms, stir, and cook for 3 minutes. Add the broccoli, and stir. Add peppers, and stir again.
3.Add the salt, pepper, pumpkin seeds, and pepper flakes, stir, and cook for a few minutes.
4.Add the spinach, stir gently, cook for a couple of minutes, divide on plates, and serve.

Nutrition: Calories: 271, Fat: 23.7, Fiber: 3.5, Carbohydrates: 14.4, Protein: 6.6

Cauliflower Polenta

Prep Time: 10 minutes **Cook Time:** 1 hour
Servings: 2

Ingredients:
1 cauliflower head, separated into florets and chopped
¼ cup hazelnuts
1 tablespoon olive oil + 2 teaspoons extra virgin olive oil
1 onion, peeled and chopped
3 cups shiitake mushrooms, chopped
4 garlic cloves, peeled
3 tablespoons nutritional yeast
½ cup water
Parsley, chopped, for serving

Directions:
1.Spread the hazelnuts on a lined baking sheet, place in an oven at 350ºF, and bake for 10 minutes.
2.Take hazelnuts out of the oven, leave to cool down, chop, and set aside.
3.Spread cauliflower florets on the baking sheet, drizzle 1 teaspoon oil, place in an oven at 400ºF, and bake for 30 minutes. In a bowl, mix oil with ½ teaspoon oil and toss to coat.
4.Put garlic cloves on aluminum foil, drizzle with ½ teaspoon oil, and wrap.
5.Spread the onion next to cauliflower and garlic on the baking sheet, place everything in an oven, and bake for 20 minutes.
6.Heat a pan with the rest of the oil over medium–high heat, add mushrooms, stir, and cook for 8 minutes. Take cauliflower out of the oven and transfer to a food processor.
7.Unwrap the garlic, peel, and add to the food processor.
8.Add onion, yeast, salt, and pepper, and blend well.
9.Divide the polenta on plates, top with mushrooms, hazelnuts, and parsley, and serve.

Nutrition: Calories: 534, Fat: 35.2, Fiber: 13.9, Carbohydrates: 52.6, Protein: 15.3

Roasted Cauliflower

Prep Time: 10 minutes **Cook Time:** 25 minutes
Servings: 6

Ingredients:
1 cauliflower head, separated into florets
Salt and ground black pepper, to taste
⅓ cup Parmesan cheese, grated
1 tablespoon fresh parsley, chopped
3 tablespoons olive oil
2 tablespoons extra virgin olive oil

Directions:
1.In a bowl, mix oil with garlic, salt, pepper, and cauliflower florets.
2.Toss to coat well, spread on a lined baking sheet, place in an oven at 450ºF and bake for 25 minutes, stirring halfway.
3.Add Parmesan cheese, parsley, stir, and cook for 5 minutes. Divide on plates and serve.

Nutrition: Calories: 119, Fat: 12.2, Fiber: 1.1, Carbohydrates: 2.5, Protein: 1.6

Mushroom and Spinach

Prep Time: 10 minutes **Cook Time:** 10 minutes
Servings: 4

Ingredients:
10 ounces spinach leaves, chopped
Salt and ground black pepper, to taste
14 ounces mushrooms, chopped
2 garlic cloves, peeled and minced
½ cup fresh parsley, chopped
1 onion, peeled and chopped
4 tablespoons olive oil
2 tablespoons balsamic vinegar

Directions:
1.Heat a pan with oil over medium–high heat, add garlic and onion, stir, and cook for 4 minutes.
2.Add mushrooms, stir, and cook for 3 minutes. Add spinach, stir, and cook for 3 minutes.
3.Add vinegar, salt, pepper, stir, and cook for 1 minute. Add parsley, stir, divide on plates, and serve.

Nutrition: Calories: 175, Fat: 14.7, Fiber: 3.4, Carbohydrates: 9.4, Protein: 5.8

Asian Side Salad

Prep Time: 30 minutes **Cook Time:** 10 minutes
Servings: 4

Ingredients:
1 cucumber, sliced thin
1 green onion, peeled and chopped
2 tablespoons coconut oil
1 packet Shiritaki noodles
1 tablespoon balsamic vinegar
1 tablespoon sesame oil
¼ teaspoon red pepper flakes
Salt and ground black pepper, to taste
1 teaspoon sesame seeds

Directions:
1.Cook noodles according to package instructions, drain, and rinse well.
2.Heat a pan with coconut oil over medium–high heat, add noodles, cover pan, and fry them for 5 minutes until crispy.
3.Transfer noodles to paper towels and drain the grease. In a bowl, mix cucumber slices with green onion, pepper flakes, vinegar, sesame oil, sesame seeds, salt, pepper, and noodles.
4.Toss to coat well, keep in the refrigerator for 30 minutes, and serve.

Nutrition: Calories: 110, Fat: 10.9, Fiber: 1.6, Carbohydrates: 4.7, Protein: 0.9

Green Beans with Vinaigrette

Prep Time: 10 minutes **Cook Time:** 12 minutes
Serving: 8

Ingredients:
2 ounces chorizo, chopped
1 garlic clove, peeled and minced
1 teaspoon lemon juice
2 teaspoons smoked paprika
½ cup coconut vinegar
4 tablespoons macadamia nut oil
¼ teaspoon coriander
Salt and ground black pepper, to taste
2 tablespoons coconut oil
2 tablespoons beef stock
2 pounds green beans

Directions:
1.In a blender, mix chorizo with salt, pepper, vinegar, garlic, lemon juice, paprika, coriander, and pulse well.
2.Add stock and the macadamia nut oil and blend again.
3.Heat a pan with the coconut oil over medium heat, add green beans and chorizo mixture, stir, and cook for 10 minutes.
4.Divide on plates and serve.

Nutrition: Calories: 159, Fat: 13.1, Fiber: 4.1, Carbohydrates: 8.8, Protein: 3.9

Braised Asian Eggplant

Prep Time: 10 minutes **Cook Time:** 15 minutes
Servings: 4

Ingredients:
1 Asian eggplant, cut into medium–sized pieces
1 onion, peeled and sliced thin
2 tablespoon vegetable oil
2 teaspoons garlic, minced
½ cup Vietnamese sauce
½ cup water
2 teaspoons chili paste
¼ cup coconut milk
4 green onions, chopped
For the Vietnamese sauce:
1 teaspoon erythritol
½ cup chicken stock
2 tablespoons fish sauce

Directions:
1.Put stock in a pan, and heat over medium heat.
2.Add erythritol, fish sauce, stir well and set aside.
3.Heat a pan over medium–high heat, add the eggplant pieces, brown them for 2 minutes, and transfer to a plate.
4.Heat the pan again with the oil over medium–high heat, add onion and garlic, stir, and cook for 2 minutes.
5.Return eggplant pieces and cook for 2 minutes.
6.Add water, Vietnamese sauce, chili paste, coconut milk, stir, and cook for 5 minutes.
7.Add green onions, stir, cook for 1 minute, transfer to plates, and serve.

Nutrition: Calories: 125, Fat: 10.9, Fiber: 1.3, Carbohydrates: 6.4, Protein: 1.7

Cheddar Soufflés

Prep Time: 10 minutes **Cook Time:** 25 minutes
Servings: 8

Ingredients:
¾ cup heavy cream
2 cups cheddar cheese, shredded
6 eggs
Salt and ground black pepper, to taste
¼ teaspoon cream of tartar
A pinch of cayenne pepper
½ teaspoon xanthan gum
1 teaspoon dry mustard
¼ cup fresh chives, chopped
½ cup almond flour
Vegetable oil cooking spray

Directions:
1.In a bowl, mix almond flour with salt, pepper, mustard, xanthan gum, cayenne, and whisk.
2.Add cheese, cream, chives, eggs, cream of tartar, and whisk again.
3.Grease 8 ramekins with cooking spray, pour the cheddar and chive mixture, place in an oven at 350ºF, bake for 25 minutes, and serve.

Nutrition: Calories: 211, Fat: 17.7, Fiber: 0.2, Carbohydrates: 1.4, Protein:11.8

Cauliflower Side Salad

Prep Time: 10 minutes **Cook Time:** 5 minutes
Servings: 10

Ingredients:
21 ounces cauliflower, separated into florets
Salt and ground black pepper, to taste
1 cup onion, chopped
1 cup celery, chopped
2 tablespoons cider vinegar
1 teaspoon erythritol
4 eggs, hard–boiled, peeled, and chopped
1 cup mayonnaise
1 tablespoon water

Directions:
1.Put cauliflower florets in a heatproof bowl, add water, cover, and cook in a microwave for 5 minutes.
2.Set aside for 5 minutes and transfer to a salad bowl.
3.Add celery, eggs, and onions, and stir gently. In a bowl, mix mayonnaise with salt, pepper, erythritol, vinegar, and whisk.
4.Add this to the salad, toss to coat well, and serve.

Nutrition: Calories: 139, Fat: 9.7, Fiber: 1.9, Carbohydrates: 10.8, Protein: 3.8

Cauliflower Rice

Prep Time: 10 minutes **Cook Time:** 30 minutes
Servings: 4

Ingredients:
1 cauliflower head, separated into florets
Salt and ground black pepper, to taste
10 ounces coconut milk
½ cup water
2 ginger slices
2 tablespoons coconut shreds, toasted

Directions:
1.Put cauliflower in a food processor and blend. Transfer cauliflower rice to a kitchen towel, press well, and set aside.
2.Heat a pot with the coconut milk over medium heat.
3.Add water and ginger, stir, and bring to a simmer. Add cauliflower, stir, and cook for 30 minutes.
4.Discard the ginger, add salt, pepper and coconut shreds, stir gently, divide on plates, and serve.

Nutrition: Calories: 223, Fat: 19.5, Fiber: 3.8, Carbohydrates: 12.4, Protein: 3.4

Snacks and Appetizers

Jalapeño Crisps

Prep Time: 10 minutes **Cook Time:** 25 minutes
Servings: 20

Ingredients:
3 tablespoons olive oil
5 jalapeños, sliced
8 ounces Parmesan cheese, grated
½ teaspoon onion powder
Salt and ground black pepper, to taste
Tabasco sauce, for serving

Directions:
1.In a bowl, mix jalapeño slices with salt, pepper, oil, and onion powder, toss to coat, and spread on a lined baking sheet.
2.Place in an oven at 450ºF and bake for 15 minutes.
3.Take jalapeño slices out of the oven, and let them cool down. In a bowl, mix pepper slices with the cheese, and press well.
4.Arrange all slices on another lined baking sheet, place in an oven again, and bake for 10 minutes.
5.Let jalapeños to cool down, arrange on a plate, and serve with Tabasco sauce on the side.

Nutrition: Calories: 56, Fat: 4.6, Fiber: 0.1, Carbohydrates: 0.6, Protein: 3.7

Cucumber Cups

Prep Time: 10 minutes **Cook Time:** 0 minutes
Servings: 24

Ingredients:
2 cucumbers, peeled, cut into ¾–inch slices, and some of the seeds scooped out
½ cup sour cream
Salt, and ground white pepper, to taste
6 ounces smoked salmon, flaked
⅓ cup fresh cilantro, chopped
2 teaspoons lime juice
1 tablespoon lime zest
A pinch of cayenne pepper

Directions:
1.In a bowl, mix salmon with salt, pepper, cayenne, sour cream, lime juice, zest, cilantro, and stir well.
2.Fill each cucumber cup with salmon mixture, arrange on a platter, and serve.

Nutrition: Calories: 22, Fat: 1.3, Fiber: 0.1, Carbohydrates: 1.1, Protein: 1.6

Caviar Salad

Prep Time: 6 minutes **Cook Time:** 0 minutes
Servings: 16

Ingredients:
8 eggs, hard–boiled, peeled, and mashed with a fork
4 ounces black caviar
4 ounces red caviar
Salt and ground black pepper, to taste
1 onion, peeled and diced
¾ cup mayonnaise

Directions:
1.In a bowl, mix mashed eggs with mayonnaise, salt, pepper, onion, and stir well.
2.Set aside for 15 minutes to cool and serve.

Nutrition: Calories: 113, Fat: 8.4, Fiber: 0.2, Carbohydrates: 4, Protein: 6.4

Cheese Fries

Prep Time: 10 minutes **Cook Time:** 5 minutes
Servings: 4

Ingredients:
1 cup marinara sauce
8 ounces queso blanco, patted dried, and sliced into fries
2 ounces tallow

Directions:
1.Heat a pan with the tallow over medium–high heat.
2.Add queso blanco pieces, cover, cook for 2 minutes on each side, and transfer to paper towels.
3.Drain excess grease, transfer them to a bowl, and serve with marinara sauce on the side.

Nutrition: Calories: 284, Fat: 23.5, Fiber: 1.6, Carbohydrates: 8.6, Protein: 8.7

Special Tortilla Chips

Prep Time: 10 minutes **Cook Time:** 14 minutes
Servings: 6

Ingredients:
For the tortillas:
2 teaspoons olive oil
1 cup flaxseed meal
2 tablespoons psyllium husk powder
¼ teaspoon xanthan gum
1 cup water
½ teaspoon curry powder
3 teaspoons coconut flour
For the chips:
6 flaxseed tortillas
Salt and ground black pepper, to taste
3 tablespoons vegetable oil
Fresh tomato paste, for serving
Sour cream, for serving

Directions:
1.In a bowl, mix flaxseed meal with psyllium powder, olive oil, xanthan gum, water, curry powder, and mix until you obtain an elastic dough.
2.Spread coconut flour on a working surface.
3.Divide dough into 6 pieces, place each piece on the work surface, roll into a circle, and cut each into 6 pieces.
4.Heat a pan with the vegetable oil over medium–high heat, add the tortilla chips, cook for 2 minutes on each side, and transfer to paper towels.
5.Put tortilla chips in a bowl, season with salt, pepper, and serve with some fresh tomato paste, and sour cream on the side.

Nutrition: Calories: 335, Fat: 18.8, Fiber: 12.6, Carbohydrates: 35.4, Protein: 8.6

Marinated Kebabs

Prep Time: 20 minutes **Cook Time:** 10 minutes
Servings: 6

Ingredients:
1 red bell pepper, seeded, and cut into chunks
1 green bell pepper, seeded, and cut into chunks
1 orange bell pepper, seeded, and cut into chunks
2 pounds sirloin steak, cut into medium–sized cubes
4 garlic cloves, peeled and minced
1 onion, peeled and cut into chunks
Salt and ground black pepper, to taste
2 tablespoons Dijon mustard
2, and ½ tablespoons Worcestershire sauce
¼ cup tamari sauce
¼ cup lemon juice
½ cup olive oil

Directions:
1.In a bowl, mix Worcestershire sauce with salt, pepper, garlic, mustard, tamari, lemon juice, oil, and whisk.
2.Add beef, bell peppers, and onion to mixture, toss to coat, and set aside for a few minutes.
3.Arrange bell pepper, meat, and onion on skewers, alternating colors, place them on a preheated grill pan over medium–high heat, cook for 5 minutes on each side, transfer to a platter, and serve.

Nutrition: Calories: 466, Fat: 26.5, Fiber: 1.4, Carbohydrates: 7.9, Protein: 48.5

Zucchini Rolls

Prep Time: 10 minutes **Cook Time:** 5 minutes
Servings: 24

Ingredients:
2 tablespoons olive oil
3 zucchini, sliced thin
24 fresh basil leaves
2 tablespoons fresh mint, chopped
1⅓ cup ricotta cheese
Salt and ground black pepper, to taste
¼ cup fresh basil, chopped

Directions:
1.Brush zucchini slices with olive oil, season with salt and pepper on both sides, place them on preheated grill pan over medium heat, cook them for 2 minutes, flip, and cook for another 2 minutes.
2.Place zucchini slices on a plate, and set aside.
3.In a bowl, mix ricotta with chopped basil, mint, salt, pepper, and stir well.
4.Spread over the zucchini slices, divide the basil leaves, roll, and serve as an appetizer.

Nutrition: Calories: 67, Fat: 4.2, Fiber: 0.3, Carbohydrates: 2.8, Protein: 4.7

Green Crackers

Prep Time: 10 minutes **Cook Time:** 24 hours
Servings: 6

Ingredients:
2 cups flaxseeds, ground
2 cups flaxseeds, soaked overnight, and drained
4 bunches kale, chopped
1 bunch fresh basil, chopped
½ bunch celery, chopped
4 garlic cloves, peeled and minced
⅓ cup olive oil

Directions:
1.In a food processor, mix ground flaxseed with celery, kale, basil, garlic, and blend well. Add oil, soaked flaxseed, and blend again.
2.Spread on a tray, cut into medium crackers, place in a dehydrator, and dry for 24 hours at 115ºF, turning them halfway.
3.Arrange them on a platter and serve.

Nutrition: Calories: 634, Fat: 43.9, Fiber: 26.8, Carbohydrates: 34.6, Protein: 21.8

Cheese and Pesto Terrine

Prep Time: 30 minutes **Cook Time:** 0 minutes
Servings: 10

Ingredients:
½ cup heavy cream
10 ounces goats cheese, crumbled
3 tablespoons basil pesto
Salt and ground black pepper, to taste
5 sundried tomatoes, cored and chopped
¼ cup pine nuts +and 1 tablespoon pine nuts, toasted and chopped

Directions:
1.In a bowl, mix goats cheese with heavy cream, salt, pepper, and stir using a mixer.
2.Spoon half of mixture into a lined bowl and spread.
3.Add pesto on top and spread this as well.
4.Add another layer of cheese, then add the sundried tomatoes and ¼ cup pine nuts.
5.Spread one final layer of cheese, and top with 1 tablespoon pine nuts.
6.Keep in the refrigerator for a couple of hours, turn upside down on a plate, and serve.

Nutrition: Calories: 173, Fat: 10.8, Fiber: 2.2, Carbohydrates: 9.8, Protein: 6.1

Avocado Salsa

Prep Time: 10 minutes **Cook Time:** 0 minutes
Servings: 4

Ingredients:
1 onion, peeled and chopped
2 avocados, pitted, peeled, and chopped
3 jalapeño pepper, chopped
Salt and ground black pepper, to taste
2 tablespoons cumin powder
2 tablespoons lime juice
½ tomato, cored and chopped

Directions:
1.In a bowl, mix onion with avocado, peppers, salt, black pepper, cumin, lime juice, tomato pieces, and stir well.
2.Transfer to a bowl and serve.

Nutrition: Calories: 221, Fat: 19.7, Fiber: 7.7, Carbohydrates: 12.1, Protein: 2.4

Pesto Crackers

Prep Time: 10 minutes **Cook Time:** 17 minutes
Servings: 6

Ingredients:
½ teaspoon baking powder
Salt and ground black pepper, to taste
1¼ cups almond flour
¼ teaspoon dried basil
1 garlic clove, peeled and minced
2 tablespoons basil pesto
A pinch of cayenne pepper
3 tablespoons butter

Directions:
1.In a bowl, mix salt, pepper, baking powder, and almond flour.
2.Add garlic, cayenne, and basil, and stir. Add pesto and whisk.
3.Add butter and mix the dough with your fingers.
4.Spread dough on a lined baking sheet, place in an oven at 325ºF, and bake for 17 minutes.
5.Set aside to cool down, cut the crackers, and serve.

Nutrition: Calories: 154, Fat: 14.9, Fiber: 1.7, Carbohydrates: 4.6, Protein: 4.2

Egg Chips

Prep Time: 5 minutes **Cook Time:** 10 minutes
Servings: 2

Ingredients:
½ tablespoon water
2 tablespoons Parmesan cheese, shredded
4 eggs whites
Salt and ground black pepper, to taste

Directions:
1.In a bowl, mix egg whites with salt, pepper, water, and whisk.
2.Spoon into a muffin pan, sprinkle cheese on top, place in an oven at 400ºF, and bake for 15 minutes.
3.Transfer egg white chips to a platter and serve.

Nutrition: Calories: 124, Fat: 6.1, Fiber: 0, Carbohydrates: 1.5, Protein: 16.2

Sausage and Cheese Dip

Prep Time: 10 minutes **Cook Time:** 2 hours and 10 minutes
Servings: 28

Ingredients:
8 ounces cream cheese
A pinch of salt, and black pepper
16 ounces sour cream
8 ounces pepper jack cheese, chopped
15 ounces canned tomatoes mixed with habaneros
1 pound Italian sausage, ground
¼ cup green onions, chopped

Directions:
1.Heat a pan over medium heat, add sausage, stir, and cook until it browns.
2.Add tomato mixture, stir, and cook for 4 minutes.
3.Add a pinch of salt and pepper and the green onions, stir, and cook for 4 minutes.
4.Spread pepper jack cheese on the bottom of a slow cooker.
5.Add the cream cheese, sausage mixture, and sour cream, cover, and cook on high for 2 hours.
6.Uncover slow cooker, stir the dip, transfer to a bowl, and serve.

Nutrition: Calories: 154, Fat: 28, Fiber: 0.2, Carbohydrates: 1.7, Protein: 6.5

Marinated Eggs

Prep Time: 2 hours and 10 minutes **Cook Time:** 7 minutes
Servings: 4

Ingredients:
6 eggs
1¼ cups water
¼ cup unsweetened rice vinegar
2 tablespoons coconut aminos
Salt and ground black pepper, to taste
2 garlic cloves, peeled and minced
1 teaspoon stevia
4 ounces cream cheese
1 tablespoon fresh chives, chopped

Directions:
1.Put eggs in a pot, add water to cover, bring to a boil over medium heat, cover, and cook for 7 minutes.
2.Rinse eggs with cold water, andset them aside to cool down.
3.In a bowl, mix 1 cup water with coconut aminos, vinegar, stevia, garlic, and whisk.
4.Put eggs in this mixture, cover with kitchen towel, and set aside for 2 hours, rotating them from time to time.
5.Peel eggs, cut in half, and put the egg yolks in a bowl.
6.Add remaining water, cream cheese, salt, pepper, chives, and stir well.
7.Stuff egg whites with mixture and serve.

Nutrition: Calories: 201, Fat: 16.5, Fiber: 0.1, Carbohydrates: 2.8, Protein: 10.6

Onion and Cauliflower Dip

Prep Time: 2 hours 10 minutes **Cook Time:** 30 minutes
Servings: 24

Ingredients:
1½ cups chicken stock
1 cauliflower head, separated into florets
¼ cup mayonnaise
½ cup onion, peeled and chopped
¾ cup cream cheese
½ teaspoon chili powder
½ teaspoon cumin
½ teaspoon garlic powder
Salt and ground black pepper, to taste

Directions:
1.Put the stock in a saucepan, add the cauliflower and onion, heat over medium heat, and cook for 30 minutes.
2.Add chili powder, salt, pepper, cumin, and garlic powder, and stir.
3.Add cream cheese, and stir a bit until it melts.
4.Blend using an immersion blender and mix with the mayonnaise.
5.Transfer to a bowl, and keep in the refrigerator for 2 hours before serving.

Nutrition: Calories: 39, Fat: 3.4, Fiber: 0.3, Carbohydrates: 1.6, Protein: 0.8

Pumpkin Muffins

Prep Time: 10 minutes **Cook Time:** 15 minutes
Servings: 18

Ingredients:
¼ cup sunflower seed butter
¾ cup pumpkin puree
2 tablespoons flaxseed meal
¼ cup coconut flour
½ cup erythritol
½ teaspoon ground nutmeg
1 teaspoon ground cinnamon
½ teaspoon baking soda
1 egg
½ teaspoon baking powder
A pinch of salt

Directions:
1.In a bowl, mix butter with the pumpkin puree, and egg and blend well.
2.Add flaxseed meal, coconut flour, erythritol, baking soda, baking powder, nutmeg, cinnamon, a pinch of salt and stir well.
3.Spoon into a greased muffin pan, place in an oven at 350ºF, and bake for 15 minutes.
4.Let the muffins cool down and serve.

Nutrition: Calories: 42, Fat: 2.6, Fiber: 1.4, Carbohydrates: 4.9, Protein: 1.6

Jalapeño Balls

Prep Time: 10 minutes **Cook Time:** 10 minutes
Servings: 3

Ingredients:
3 bacon slices
3 ounces cream cheese
¼ teaspoon onion powder
Salt and ground black pepper, to taste
1 jalapeño pepper, chopped
½ teaspoon dried parsley
¼ teaspoon garlic powder

Directions:
1.Heat a pan over medium–high heat, add bacon, cook until crispy, transfer to paper towels, drain grease, and crumble.
2.Reserve bacon fat from the pan.
3.In a bowl, mix cream cheese with jalapeño pepper, onion powder, garlic powder, parsley, salt, pepper, and stir well.
4.Add bacon fat and crumbled bacon, stir gently, shape balls from this mixture, and serve.

Nutrition: Calories: 205, Fat: 17.9, Fiber: 0.2, Carbohydrates: 1.6, Protein: 9.3

Cheeseburger Muffins

Prep Time: 10 minutes **Cook Time:** 30 minutes
Servings: 9

Ingredients:
½ cup flaxseed meal
½ cup almond flour
Salt and ground black pepper, to taste
2 eggs
1 teaspoon baking powder
¼ cups sour cream
For the filling:
½ teaspoon onion powder
16 ounces ground beef
Salt and ground black pepper, to taste
2 tablespoons tomato paste
½ teaspoon garlic powder
½ cup cheddar cheese, grated
2 tablespoons mustard

Directions:
1.In a bowl, mix almond flour with flaxseed meal, salt, pepper, baking powder, and whisk. Add eggs, sour cream, and stir well.
2.Divide into a greased muffin pan and press well using your fingers.
3.Heat a pan over medium–high heat, add beef, stir, and brown for a few minutes.
4.Add salt, pepper, onion powder, garlic powder, tomato paste, and stir well. Cook for 5 minutes and take off the heat.
5.Fill the cupcakes crusts with this mixture, place in an oven at 350ºF, and bake for 15 minutes.
6.Spread cheese on top, place in an oven again, and bake muffins for 5 minutes. Serve warm.

Nutrition: Calories: 203, Fat: 9, Fiber: 2.4, Carbohydrates: 4.4, Protein: 20.5

Pizza Dip

Prep Time: 10 minutes **Cook Time:** 20 minutes
Servings: 4

Ingredients:
4 ounces cream cheese, softened
½ cup mozzarella cheese
¼ cup sour cream
Salt and ground black pepper, to taste
½ cup tomato sauce
¼ cup mayonnaise
¼ cup Parmesan cheese, grated
1 tablespoon green bell pepper, seeded and chopped
6 pepperoni slices, chopped
½ teaspoon Italian seasoning
4 black olives, pitted and chopped

Directions:
1.In a bowl, mix cream cheese with mozzarella cheese, sour cream, mayonnaise, salt, pepper, and stir well.
2.Spread into 4 ramekins, add a layer of tomato sauce, then layer Parmesan cheese, and top with bell pepper, pepperoni, Italian seasoning, and black olives.
3.Place in an oven at 350ºF and bake for 20 minutes. Serve warm.

Nutrition: Calories: 284, Fat: 24.4, Fiber: 1, Carbohydrates: 9.5, Protein: 8.6

Flaxseed and Almond Muffins

Prep Time: 10 minutes **Cook Time:** 15 minutes
Servings: 20

Ingredients:
½ cup flaxseed meal
½ cup almond flour
3 tablespoons swerve
1 tablespoon psyllium powder
A pinch of salt
Vegetable oil cooking spray
¼ teaspoon baking powder
1 egg
¼ cup coconut milk
⅓ cup sour cream
4 hot dogs, cut into 20 pieces

Directions:
1.In a bowl, mix flaxseed meal with flour, psyllium powder, swerve, salt, baking powder, and stir.
2.Add egg, sour cream, coconut milk, and whisk.
3.Grease a muffin tray with cooking oil, divide this batter, place a hot dog piece in the middle of each muffin, place in an oven at 350ºF, and bake for 12 minutes.
4.Broil in preheated broiler for 3 minutes, divide on a platter, and serve.

Nutrition: Calories: 65, Fat: 3.4, Fiber: 0.9, Carbohydrates: 7.1, Protein: 1.7

Fried Queso

Prep Time: 10 minutes **Cook Time:** 10 minutes
Servings: 6

Ingredients:
2 ounces olives, pitted and chopped
5 ounces queso blanco, cubed and slightly frozen
A pinch of red pepper flakes
1½ tablespoons olive oil

Directions:
1.Heat a pan with the oil over medium–high heat, add queso cubes, and cook until bottom melts a bit.
2.Flip cubes with a spatula, and sprinkle black olives on top.
3.Let the cubes cook a bit more, flip again, sprinkle with red pepper flakes, and cook until crispy.
4.Flip, cook on the other side until crispy, transfer to a cutting board, cut into small blocks, and serve.

Nutrition: Calories: 152, Fat: 15.8, Fiber: 0.3, Carbohydrates: 0.6, Protein: 3.2

Maple and Pecan Bars

Prep Time: 10 minutes **Cook Time:** 25 minutes
Servings: 12

Ingredients:
½ cup flaxseed meal
2 cups pecans, toasted, and crushed
1 cup almond flour
½ cup coconut oil
¼ teaspoon stevia
½ cup coconut, shredded
¼ cup "maple syrup"
For the maple syrup:
¼ cup erythritol
2¼ teaspoons coconut oil
1 tablespoon butter
¼ teaspoon xanthan gum
¾ cup water
2 teaspoons maple extract
½ teaspoon vanilla extract

Directions:
1.In a heatproof bowl, mix butter with 2¼ teaspoons coconut oil, xanthan gum, stir, place in a microwave, and heat up for 1 minute.
2.Add erythritol, water, maple, vanilla extract, stir well, and heat in a microwave for 1 minute. In a bowl, mix the flaxseed meal with coconut and almond flour, and stir.
3.Add pecans and stir again. Add ¼ cup "maple syrup," stevia, ½ cup coconut oil, and stir well.
4.Spread in a baking dish, press well, place in an oven at 350ºF, and bake for 25 minutes.
5.Set aside to cool down, cut into 12 bars, and serve.

Nutrition: Calories: 313, Fat: 31.1, Fiber: 3, Carbohydrates: 11.8, Protein: 2.7

Pepperoni Bombs

Prep Time: 10 minutes **Cook Time:** 0 minutes
Servings: 6

Ingredients:
8 black olives, pitted and chopped
Salt and ground black pepper, to taste
2 tablespoons sundried tomato pesto
14 pepperoni slices, chopped
4 ounces cream cheese
1 tablespoon fresh basil, chopped

Directions:
1.In a bowl, mix cream cheese with salt, pepper, pepperoni, basil, sundried tomato pesto, black olives, and stir well.
2.Shape balls from mixture, arrange on a platter, and serve.

Nutrition: Calories: 140, Fat: 6, Fiber: 0.3, Carbohydrates: 1.2, Protein: 4.5

Zucchini Chips

Prep Time: 10 minutes **Cook Time:** 3 hours
Servings: 8

Ingredients:
3 zucchini, sliced thin
Salt and ground black pepper, to taste
2 tablespoons olive oil
2 tablespoons balsamic vinegar

Directions:
1.In a bowl, mix the oil with vinegar, salt, pepper, and whisk.
2.Add the zucchini slices, toss to coat well, and spread on a lined baking sheet, place in an oven at 200ºF and bake for 3 hours.
3.Let the chips to cool down and serve.

Nutrition: Calories: 43, Fat: 3.6, Fiber: 0.8, Carbohydrates: 2.5, Protein: 0.9

Simple Tomato Tarts

Prep Time: 10 minutes **Cook Time:** 1 hour and 10 minutes
Servings: 12

Ingredients:
¼ cup olive oil
2 tomatoes, cored and sliced
Salt and ground black pepper, to taste
For the base:
5 tablespoons butter
1 tablespoon psyllium husk
½ cup almond flour
2 tablespoons coconut flour
A pinch of salt
For the filling:
2 teaspoons garlic, minced
3 teaspoons fresh thyme, chopped
2 tablespoons olive oil
3 ounces goats cheese, crumbled
1 small onion, sliced thin

Directions:
1.Spread tomato slices on a lined baking sheet, season with salt, pepper, drizzle ¼ cup olive oil, place in an oven at 425ºF and bake for 40 minutes.
2.In a food processor, mix almond flour with psyllium husk, coconut flour, salt, pepper, and cold butter, and stir until you obtain a dough.
3.Divide dough into silicone cupcake molds, press well, place in an oven at 350ºF and bake for 20 minutes.
4.Take cupcakes out of the oven and set aside.
5.Take tomato slices out of the oven and let them cool briefly.
6.Divide tomato slices on top of cupcakes.
7.Heat a pan with 2 tablespoons olive oil over medium–high heat, add onion, stir, and cook for 4 minutes.
8.Add garlic and thyme, stir, cook for 1 minute, and take off heat.
9.Spread mixture on top of tomato slices.
10.Sprinkle with goats cheese, place in an oven again, and cook at 350ºF for 5 minutes. Arrange on a platter and serve.

Nutrition: Calories: 125, Fat: 11.7, Fiber: 3.1, Carbohydrates: 5.1, Protein: 0.9

Baked Chia Seeds

Prep Time: 10 minutes **Cook Time:** 35 minutes **Servings:** 36

Ingredients:
1¼ cup ice water
½ cup chia seeds, ground
3 ounces cheddar, cheese, grated
¼ teaspoon xanthan gum
2 tablespoons olive oil
2 tablespoons psyllium husk powder
¼ teaspoon dried oregano
¼ teaspoon garlic powder
¼ teaspoon onion powder
Salt and ground black pepper, to taste
¼ teaspoon sweet paprika

Directions:
1.In a bowl, mix chia seeds with xanthan gum, psyllium powder, oregano, garlic, onion powder, paprika, salt, pepper, and stir.
2.Add oil and stir well. Add ice water and stir until you obtain a firm dough.
3.Spread this on a baking sheet, place in an oven at 350ºF, and bake for 35 minutes.
4.Set aside to cool down, cut into 36 crackers, and serve.

Nutrition: Calories: 11, Fat: 1, Fiber: 0, Carbohydrates: 0.1, Protein: 0.6

Avocado Dip

Prep Time: 3 hours and 10 minutes **Cook Time:** 10 minutes **Servings:** 4

Ingredients:
¼ cup erythritol powder
2 avocados, pitted, peeled, and cut into slices
¼ teaspoon stevia
½ cup fresh cilantro, chopped
Juice, and zest of 2 limes
1 cup coconut milk

Directions:
1.Place the avocado slices on a lined baking sheet, squeeze half the lime juice over them, and keep in a freezer for 3 hours.
2.Heat the coconut milk in a pan over medium heat.
3.Add lime zest, stir, and bring to a boil.
4.Add erythritol powder, stir, take off heat, and set aside to cool.
5.Transfer avocado to a food processor, add rest of the lime juice, and the cilantro, and pulse well.
6.Add coconut milk mixture, stevia, and blend well. Transfer to a bowl and serve.

Nutrition: Calories: 352, Fat: 33.9, Fiber: 8.1, Carbohydrates: 17.3, Protein: 3.3

Prosciutto–wrapped Shrimp

Prep Time: 10 minutes **Cook Time:** 20 minutes **Servings:** 16

Ingredients:
2 tablespoons olive oil
10 ounces already cooked shrimp, peeled and deveined
1 tablespoonsfresh mint, chopped
2 tablespoons erythritol
⅓ cup blackberries, mashed
11 prosciutto sliced
⅓ cup red wine

Directions:
1.Wrap each shrimp in prosciutto slices, arrange on a lined baking sheet, drizzle olive oil over them, place in an oven at 425ºF, and bake for 15 minutes.
2.Heat a pan with mashed blackberries over medium heat, add mint, wine, and erythritol, stir, cook for 3 minutes, and take off heat.
3.Arrange shrimp on a platter, drizzle blackberries sauce over them, and serve.

Nutrition: Calories: 89, Fat: 5.5, Fiber: 0.2, Carbohydrates: 1.1, Protein: 10.1

Broccoli and Cheddar Biscuits

Prep Time: 10 minutes **Cook Time:** 25 minutes
Servings: 12

Ingredients:
4 cups broccoli florets
1½ cup almond flour
1 teaspoon paprika
Salt and ground black pepper, to taste
2 eggs
¼ cup coconut oil
2 cups cheddar cheese, grated
1 teaspoon garlic powder
½ teaspoon apple cider vinegar
½ teaspoon baking soda

Directions:
1.Put broccoli florets in a food processor, add some salt and pepper, and blend well.
2.In a bowl, mix almond flour with salt, pepper, paprika, garlic powder, baking soda, and stir.
3.Add cheddar cheese, coconut oil, eggs, and vinegar, and stir. Add broccoli, and stir again.
4.Shape 12 patties, arrange on a baking sheet, place in an oven at 375ºF, and bake for 20 minutes.
5.Turn oven to broiler, and broil the biscuits for 5 minutes. Arrange on a platter and serve.

Nutrition: Calories: 210, Fat: 18.1, Fiber: 2.3, Carbohydrates: 5.3, Protein: 9.3

Corndogs

Prep Time: 10 minutes **Cook Time:** 10 minutes
Servings: 4

Ingredients:
1½ cups olive oil
2 tablespoons heavy cream
1 cup almond meal
4 sausages
1 teaspoon baking powder
1 teaspoon Italian seasoning
2 eggs
½ teaspoon turmeric
Salt and ground black pepper, to taste
A pinch of cayenne pepper

Directions:
1.In a bowl, mix almond meal with Italian seasoning, baking powder, turmeric, salt, pepper, cayenne, and stir well.
2.In another bowl, mix eggs with heavy cream, and whisk.
3.Combine the 2 mixtures and stir well.
4.Dip sausages in mixture, and place them on a plate.
5.Heat a pan with oil over medium–high heat, add the sausages, cook for 2 minutes on each side, and transfer to paper towels.
6.Drain grease, arrange on a platter, and serve.

Nutrition: Calories: 980, Fat: 103.9, Fiber: 3, Carbohydrates: 5.5, Protein: 15.8

Saucy Zucchini

Prep Time: 10 minutes **Cook Time:** 15 minutes
Servings: 4

Ingredients:
1 cup mozzarella cheese, shredded
¼ cup tomato sauce
1 zucchini, sliced
Salt and ground black pepper, to taste
A pinch of cumin
Vegetable oil cooking spray

Directions:
1.Spray a cooking sheet with some oil and arrange zucchini slices on it.
2.Spread the tomato sauce all over zucchini slices, season with salt, pepper, cumin, and sprinkle with shredded mozzarella.
3.Place in an oven at 350ºF and bake for 15 minutes. Arrange on a platter, and serve.

Nutrition: Calories: 32, Fat: 1.4, Fiber: 0.8, Carbohydrates: 2.7, Protein: 2.8

Simple Hummus

Prep Time: 10 minutes **Cook Time:** 0 minutes
Servings: 5

Ingredients:
4 cups zucchini, diced
¼ cup olive oil
Salt and ground black pepper, to taste
4 garlic cloves, peeled and minced
¾ cup tahini
½ cup lemon juice
1 tablespoon cumin

Directions:
1.In a blender, mix zucchini with salt, pepper, oil, lemon juice, garlic, tahini, and cumin, and blend well.
2.Transfer to a bowl and serve.

Nutrition: Calories: 329, Fat: 30.1, Fiber: 4.6, Carbohydrates: 12.5, Protein: 7.8

Mini Bell Pepper Nachos

Prep Time: 10 minutes **Cook Time:** 20 minutes
Servings: 6

Ingredients:
1 pound mini bell peppers, seeded and cut into halves
Salt and ground black pepper, to taste
1 teaspoon garlic powder
1 teaspoon sweet paprika
½ teaspoon dried oregano
¼ teaspoon red pepper flakes
1 pound ground beef
1½ cups cheddar cheese, shredded
1 tablespoons chili powder
1 teaspoon cumin
½ cup tomato, cored and chopped
Sour cream, for serving

Directions:
1.In a bowl, mix chili powder with paprika, salt, pepper, cumin, oregano, pepper flakes, garlic powder, and stir.
2.Heat a pan over medium heat, add beef, stir, and brown for 10 minutes. Add chili powder mixture, stir, and take off the heat.
3.Arrange pepper halves on a lined baking sheet, stuff them with the beef mixture, sprinkle with cheese, place in an oven at 400ºF, and bake for 10 minutes.
4.Take peppers out of the oven, sprinkle with the tomatoes, divide on plates, and serve with sour cream on top.

Nutrition: Calories: 581, Fat: 39.2, Fiber: 1.9, Carbohydrates: 6.5, Protein: 49.7

Almond Butter Bars

Prep Time: 2 hours and 10 minutes **Cook Time:** 2 minutes
Servings: 12

Ingredients:
¾ cup coconut, unsweetened and shredded
¾ cup almond butter
¾ cup stevia
1 cup almond butter
2 tablespoons almond butter
4. 5 ounces dark chocolate, chopped
2 tablespoons coconut oil

Directions:
1.In a bowl, mix almond flour with stevia and coconut, and stir well.
2.Heat a pan over medium–low heat, add 1 cup almond butter and coconut oil, and whisk.
3.Add to almond flour and stir well. Transfer to a baking dish and press well. Heat another pan with the chocolate, stirring often.
4.Add rest of the almond butter and whisk again.
5.Pour over almond mixture, and spread evenly. Place in the refrigerator for 2 hours, cut into 12 bars, and serve.

Nutrition: Calories: 184, Fat: 12.7, Fiber: 2.9, Carbohydrates: 14.6, Protein: 5.7

Beef Jerky

Prep Time: 6 hours **Cook Time:** 4 hours
Servings: 6

Ingredients:
2 cups soy sauce
½ cup Worcestershire sauce
2 tablespoons black peppercorns
2 tablespoons ground black pepper
2 pounds beef round, sliced

Directions:
1.In a bowl, mix soy sauce with black peppercorns, black pepper, Worcestershire sauce, and whisk.
2.Add beef slices, toss to coat, and set aside in the refrigerator for 6 hours.
3.Spread on a rack, place in an oven at 370ºF, and bake for 4 hours. Transfer to a bowl and serve.

Nutrition: Calories: 455, Fat: 9.8, Fiber: 0.7, Carbohydrates: 10.5, Protein: 76

Celery Sticks

Prep Time: 10 minutes **Cook Time:** 0 minutes
Servings: 12

Ingredients:
2 cups rotisserie chicken, shredded
6 celery stalks, cut into halves
3 tablespoons tomato sauce
¼ cup mayonnaise
Salt and ground black pepper, to taste
½ teaspoon garlic powder
Some chopped chives, for serving

Directions:
1.In a bowl, mix chicken with salt, pepper, garlic powder, mayonnaise, tomato sauce, and stir well.
2.Arrange celery pieces on a platter, spread chicken mixture over them, sprinkle some chives, and serve.

Nutrition: Calories: 75, Fat: 2, Fiber: 0.2, Carbohydrates: 2.6, Protein: 11.8

Garlic Spinach Dip

Prep Time: 10 minutes **Cook Time:** 35 minutes
Servings: 6

Ingredients:
6 bacon slices
5 ounces spinach
½ cup sour cream
8 ounces cream cheese, softened
1½ tablespoons fresh parsley, chopped
2. 5 ounces Parmesan cheese, grated
Salt and ground black pepper, to taste
1 tablespoon garlic, minced

Directions:
1.Heat a pan over medium heat, add bacon, cook until crispy, transfer to paper towels, drain grease, crumble, and set aside in a bowl.
2.Heat the same pan with the bacon grease over medium heat, add spinach, stir, cook for 2 minutes, and transfer to a bowl.
3.In another bowl, mix the cream cheese with garlic, salt, pepper, sour cream, and parsley, and stir well.
4.Add bacon and stir again. Add lemon juice, spinach, and stir. Add Parmesan cheese and stir again.
5.Divide into ramekins, place in an oven at 350ºF, and bake for 25 minutes.
6.Turn the oven to broil and broil for 4 minutes. Serve with crackers.

Nutrition: Calories: 358, Fat: 30.3, Fiber: 0.6, Carbohydrates: 4, Protein: 18.9

Broccoli Sticks

Prep Time: 10 minutes **Cook Time:** 20 minutes
Servings: 20

Ingredients:
1 egg
2 cups broccoli florets
⅓ cup cheddar cheese, grated
¼ cup onion, peeled and chopped
½ cup cauliflower rice
2 tablespoons fresh parsley, chopped
A drizzle of olive oil for greasing
Salt and ground black pepper, to taste

Directions:
1.Heat a saucepan with water over medium heat, add broccoli, steam for 1 minute, drain, chop, and put into a bowl.
2.Add egg, cheddar cheese, cauliflower rice, salt, pepper, parsley, and stir well.
3.Shape sticks out of mixture using your hands and place them on a greased baking sheet.
4.Place in an oven at 400ºF and bake for 20 minutes. Arrange on a platter and serve.

Nutrition: Calories: 19, Fat: 1, Fiber: 0.3, Carbohydrates: 1.3, Protein: 1.3

Spinach Balls

Prep Time: 10 minutes **Cook Time:** 12 minutes
Servings: 30

Ingredients:
4 tablespoons melted butter
2 eggs
1 cup almond flour
16 ounces spinach
⅓ cup feta cheese, crumbled
¼ teaspoon ground nutmeg
⅓ cup Parmesan cheese, grated
Salt and ground black pepper, to taste
1 tablespoon onion powder
3 tablespoons whipping cream
1 teaspoon garlic powder

Directions:
1.In a blender, mix spinach with butter, eggs, almond flour, feta cheese, Parmesan cheese, nutmeg, whipping cream, salt, pepper, onion, garlic pepper, and blend well.
2.Transfer to a bowl and keep in the freezer for 10 minutes.
3.Shape 30 spinach balls, arrange them on a lined baking sheet, place in an oven at 350ºF, and bake for 12 minutes.
4.Let the spinach balls to cool down and serve.

Nutrition: Calories: 40, Fat: 3.5, Fiber: 0.5, Carbohydrates: 1, Protein: 1.7

Stuffed Mushrooms

Prep Time: 10 minutes **Cook Time:** 20 minutes
Servings: 5

Ingredients:
¼ cup mayonnaise
1 teaspoon garlic powder
1 onion, peeled and chopped
24 ounces white mushroom caps
Salt and ground black pepper, to taste
1 teaspoon curry powder
4 ounces cream cheese, softened
¼ cup sour cream
½ cup queso blanco or Monterey Jack cheese, shredded
1 cup shrimp, cooked, peeled, deveined, and chopped

Directions:
1.In a bowl, mix mayonnaise with garlic powder, onion, curry powder, cream cheese, sour cream, Mexican cheese, shrimp, salt and pepper to taste, and whisk.
2.Stuff mushrooms with mixture, place on a baking sheet, and cook in the oven at 350ºF for 20 minutes.
3.Arrange on a platter and serve.

Nutrition: Calories: 259, Fat: 16.8, Fiber: 1.9, Carbohydrates: 10.7, Protein: 17.6

Crab Dip

Prep Time: 10 minutes **Cook Time:** 30 minutes
Servings: 8

Ingredients:
8 bacon strips, sliced
12 ounces crab meat
½ cup mayonnaise
½ cup sour cream
8 ounces cream cheese
2 poblano pepper, seeded, and chopped
2 tablespoons lemon juice
Salt and ground black pepper, to taste
4 garlic cloves, peeled and minced
4 green onions, minced
½ cup Parmesan cheese+ ½ cup Parmesan cheese, grated
Salt and ground black pepper, to taste

Directions:
1.Heat a pan over medium–high heat, add bacon, cook until crispy, transfer to paper towels, chop, and set aside to cool down.
2.In a bowl, mix the sour cream with cream cheese and mayonnaise, and stir well.
3.Add ½ cup Parmesan cheese, poblano peppers, bacon, green onion, garlic, lemon juice, and stir again.
4.Add crab meat, salt, pepper, and stir gently.
5.Pour into a heatproof baking dish, spread rest of the Parmesan cheese, place in an oven, bake at 350ºF for 20 minutes, and serve.

Nutrition: Calories: 300, Fat: 23.7, Fiber: 0.4, Carbohydrates: 8.2, Protein: 13.2

Breadsticks

Prep Time: 10 minutes **Cook Time:** 15 minutes
Servings: 24

Ingredients:
3 tablespoons cream cheese, softened
1 tablespoon psyllium powder
¾ cup almond flour
2 cups mozzarella cheese, melted for 30 seconds in the microwave
1 teaspoon baking powder
1 egg
2 tablespoons Italian seasoning
Salt and ground black pepper, to taste
3 ounces cheddar cheese, grated
1 teaspoon onion powder

Directions:
1.In a bowl, mix psyllium powder with almond flour, baking powder, salt, pepper, and whisk.
2.Add cream cheese, melted mozzarella cheese, egg, and stir using your hands until you obtain a dough.
3.Spread on a baking sheet and cut into 24 sticks. Sprinkle with onion powder and Italian seasoning over them.
4.Top with cheddar cheese, place in an oven at 350ºF, bake for 15 minutes, and serve.

Nutrition: Calories: 35, Fat: 2.7, Fiber: 0.4, Carbohydrates: 0.9, Protein: 2.1

Italian Meatballs

Prep Time: 10 minutes **Cook Time:** 6 minutes
Servings: 16

Ingredients:
1 egg
Salt and ground black pepper, to taste
¼ cup almond flour
1 pound ground turkey
½ teaspoon garlic powder
2 tablespoons sundried tomatoes, cored and chopped
½ cup mozzarella cheese, shredded
2 tablespoons olive oil
2 tablespoon fresh basil, chopped

Directions:
1.In a bowl, mix turkey with salt, pepper, egg, almond flour, garlic powder, sundried tomatoes, mozzarella, basil, and stir well.
2.Shape 12 meatballs, heat a pan with oil over medium–high heat, drop meatballs, and cook them for 2 minutes on each side. Arrange on a platter and serve.

Nutrition: Calories: 81, Fat: 5.5, Fiber: 0.1, Carbohydrates: 0.5, Protein: 8.5

Parmesan Wings

Prep Time: 10 minutes **Cook Time:** 24 minutes **Servings:** 6

Ingredients:
6–pound chicken wings, cut in half
Salt and ground black pepper, to taste
½ teaspoon Italian seasoning
2 tablespoons butter
½ cup Parmesan cheese, grated
A pinch of red pepper flakes
1 teaspoon garlic powder
1 egg

Directions:
1.Arrange chicken wings on a lined baking sheet, place in an oven at 425ºF, and bake for 17 minutes.
2.In a blender, mix the butter with cheese, egg, salt, pepper, pepper flakes, garlic powder, Italian seasoning, and blend well.
3.Take chicken wings out of the oven, flip them, turn oven to broil, and broil them for 5 minutes.
4.Take chicken pieces out of the oven again, pour sauce, toss to coat well, broil for 1 minute, and serve.

Nutrition: Calories: 677, Fat: 50.1, Fiber: 0, Carbohydrates: 0.1, Protein: 54.2

Cheese Sticks

Prep Time: 1 hour and 10 minutes **Cook Time:** 20 minutes **Servings:** 16

Ingredients:
2 eggs, whisked
Salt and ground black pepper, to taste
8 mozzarella string cheese pieces, cut in half
1 cup Parmesan cheese, grated
1 tablespoon Italian seasoning
½ cup olive oil
1 garlic clove, peeled and minced

Directions:
1.In a bowl, mix Parmesan cheese with salt, pepper, Italian seasoning, garlic, and stir well.
2.Put whisked eggs in another bowl. Dip mozzarella sticks in egg mixture, then in the cheese mixture.
3.Dip again in the egg mixture, then in Parmesan cheese mixture, and keep in the freezer for 1 hour.
4.Heat a pan with the oil over medium–high heat, add cheese sticks, fry them until they are golden on one side, flip, and cook them the same way on the other side.
5.Arrange them on a platter and serve.

Nutrition: Calories: 116, Fat: 10.4, Fiber: 0, Carbohydrates: 0.8, Protein: 5.8

Bacon Delight

Prep Time: 15 minutes **Cook Time:** 1 hour and 20 minutes **Servings:** 16

Ingredients:
½ teaspoon ground cinnamon
2 tablespoons erythritol
16 bacon slices
1 tablespoon coconut oil
3 ounces dark chocolate
1 teaspoon maple extract

Directions:
1.In a bowl, mix cinnamon with the erythritol and stir.
2.Arrange bacon slices on a lined baking sheet and sprinkle cinnamon mixture over them.
3.Flip bacon slices and sprinkle the cinnamon mixture over them.
4.Place in an oven at 275ºF and bake for 1 hour.
5.Heat a pot with the oil over medium heat, add chocolate, and stir until it melts.
6.Add maple extract, stir, take off heat, and set aside to cool.
7.Take bacon strips out of the oven, let them cool down, dip each in chocolate mixture, place them on a parchment paper, and let them cool down completely. Serve cold.

Nutrition: Calories: 139, Fat: 10.4, Fiber: 0.2, Carbohydrates: 3.5, Protein: 7.5

Taco Cups

Prep Time: 10 minutes **Cook Time:** 40 minutes **Servings:** 30

Ingredients:
1 pound ground beef
2 cups cheddar cheese, shredded
¼ cup water
Salt and ground black pepper, to taste
2 tablespoons cumin
2 tablespoons chili powder
Pico de gallo, for serving

Directions:
1.Divide spoonfuls of cheddar cheese on a lined baking sheet, place in an oven at 350ºF, and bake for 7 minutes.
2.Let cheese cool down for 1 minute, transfer them to mini cupcake molds, and shape them into cups.
3.Heat a pan over medium–high heat, add beef, stir, and cook until it browns.
4.Add water, salt, pepper, cumin, chili powder, stir, and cook for 5 minutes.
5.Divide into cheese cups, top with pico de gallo, transfer to a platter, and serve.

Nutrition: Calories: 58, Fat: 3.4, Fiber: 0, Carbohydrates: 0.1, Protein: 6.5

Chili Lime Chips

Prep Time: 10 minutes **Cook Time:** 20 minutes **Servings:** 4

Ingredients:
1 cup almond flour
Salt and ground black pepper, to taste
1½ teaspoons lime zest
1 teaspoon lime juice
1 egg

Directions:
1.In a bowl, mix almond flour with lime zest, lime juice, salt, and stir. Add egg and whisk again.
2.Divide into 4 parts, roll each into a ball, and then spread well using a rolling pin.
3.Cut each into 6 triangles, place them on a lined baking sheet, place in an oven at 350ºF, and bake for 20 minutes.

Nutrition: Calories: 48, Fat: 3.7, Fiber: 0.9, Carbohydrates: 2, Protein: 2.6

Chicken Egg Rolls

Prep Time: 2 hours and 10 minutes **Cook Time:** 15 minutes **Servings:** 12

Ingredients:
4 ounces blue cheese
2 cups chicken, cooked, and diced
Salt and ground black pepper, to taste
2 green onions, chopped
2 celery stalks, diced
½ cup tomato sauce
½ teaspoon erythritol
For egg roll wrappers:
3 eggs, beaten 3/4 cup cold water
1 teaspoon salt
4 cups coconut flour
5 tablespoons olive oil

Directions:
1.For wrappers, mix all the ingredients.
2.Heat a wok over medium–high heat, thinly coat with olive oil, pour 1/12 of the egg mixture in approximately 7 inch circle.
3.Cook 1 minute, remove from heat, repeat with remaining mixture.
4.In a bowl, mix chicken meat with blue cheese, salt, pepper, green onions, celery, tomato sauce, and sweetener, stir well, and keep in the refrigerator for 2 hours.
5.Place egg wrappers on a working surface, divide chicken mixture on them, roll, and seal edges.
6.Heat a pan with vegetable oil over medium–high heat, add egg rolls, cook until they are golden, flip, and cook on the other side as well.
7.Arrange on a platter and serve them.

Nutrition: Calories: 156, Fat: 11, Fiber: 1.7, Carbohydrates: 3.4, Protein: 10.9

Artichoke Dip

Prep Time: 10 minutes **Cook Time:** 15 minutes
Servings: 16

Ingredients:
¼ cup sour cream
¼ cup heavy cream
¼ cup mayonnaise
¼ cup shallot, peeled and chopped
1 tablespoon olive oil
2 garlic cloves, peeled and minced
4 ounces cream cheese
½ cup Parmesan cheese, grated
1 cup mozzarella cheese, shredded
4 ounces feta cheese, crumbled
1 tablespoon balsamic vinegar
28 ounces canned artichoke hearts, chopped
Salt and ground black pepper, to taste
10 ounces spinach, chopped

Directions:
1.Heat a pan with the oil over medium heat, add shallot and garlic, stir, and cook for 3 minutes.
2.Add heavy cream and cream cheese, and stir.
3.Add sour cream, Parmesan cheese, mayonnaise, feta cheese, mozzarella cheese, stir, and reduce heat.
4.Add artichoke, spinach, salt, pepper, vinegar, stir well, take off the heat, transfer to a bowl, and serve.

Nutrition: Calories: 144, Fat: 12, Fiber: 2, Carbohydrates: 5, Protein: 5

Fish and Seafood

Tuna and Chimichurri Sauce

Prep Time: 10 minutes **Cook Time:** 5 minutes
Servings: 4

Ingredients:
½ cup fresh cilantro, chopped
⅓ cup olive oil
2 tablespoons olive oil
1 onion, peeled and chopped
3 tablespoon balsamic vinegar
2 tablespoons fresh parsley, chopped
2 tablespoons fresh basil, chopped
1 jalapeño pepper, chopped
1 pound sushi–grade tuna steak
Salt and ground black pepper, to taste
1 teaspoon red pepper flakes
1 teaspoon fresh thyme, chopped
A pinch of cayenne pepper
3 garlic cloves, peeled and minced
2 avocados, pitted, peeled, and sliced
6 ounces baby arugula

Directions:
1.In a bowl, mix ⅓ cup oil with jalapeño, vinegar, onion, cilantro, basil, garlic, parsley, pepper flakes, thyme, cayenne, salt, pepper, whisk, and set aside.
2.Heat a pan with remaining oil over medium–high heat, add tuna, season with salt, pepper, cook for 2 minutes on each side, transfer to a cutting board, set aside to cool, and slice.
3.Mix arugula with half of the chimichurri mixture and toss to coat.
4.Divide arugula on plates, top with tuna slices, drizzle the rest of the chimichurri sauce, and serve with avocado slices on the side.

Nutrition: Calories: 564, Fat: 37.6, Fiber: 8.2, Carbohydrates: 13.8, Protein: 48.6

Salmon Bites with Chili Sauce

Prep Time: 10 minutes **Cook Time:** 15 minutes
Servings: 6

Ingredients:
1¼ cups coconut, desiccated, and unsweetened
1 pound salmon, skinless and cubed
1 egg
Salt and ground black pepper, to taste
1 tablespoon water
⅓ cup coconut flour
3 tablespoons coconut oil
For the sauce:
¼ teaspoon agar
3 garlic cloves, peeled and chopped
¾ cup water
4 red chili peppers, chopped
¼ cup balsamic vinegar
½ cup stevia
A pinch of salt

Directions:
1.In a bowl, mix flour with salt, pepper, and stir. In another bowl, whisk egg and 1 tablespoon water. Put coconut in a third bowl.
2.Dip salmon cubes in flour, then in egg, and finally in desiccated coconut, and place on a plate.
3.Heat a pan with coconut oil over medium–high heat, add salmon bites, cook for 3 minutes on each side, and transfer to paper towels.
4.Heat a pan with ¾ cup water over high heat, sprinkle with the agar, and bring to a boil.
5.Cook for 3 minutes and take off heat. In a blender, mix garlic with chilies, vinegar, stevia, and a pinch of salt, and blend well.
6.Transfer to a small pan, and heat over medium–high heat.
7.Stir, add agar mixture, cook for 3 minutes. Serve salmon bites with chili sauce on the side.

Nutrition: Calories: 342, Fat: 25.8, Fiber: 6.8, Carbohydrates: 11.7, Protein: 18.3

Italian Clams Delight

Prep Time: 10 minutes **Cook Time:** 10 minutes
Servings: 6

Ingredients:
½ cup butter
36 clams, scrubbed
1 teaspoon red pepper flakes
1 teaspoon fresh parsley, chopped
5 garlic cloves, peeled and minced
1 tablespoon dried oregano
2 cups white wine

Directions:
1.Heat a pan with butter over medium heat, add garlic, stir, and cook for 1 minute.
2.Add parsley, oregano, wine, pepper flakes, and stir well.
3.Add clams, stir, cover, and cook for 10 minutes.
4.Discard any unopened clams, ladle clam mixture into bowls, and serve.

Nutrition: Calories: 287, Fat: 15.8, Fiber: 1, Carbohydrates: 21.6, Protein: 1.5

Sardine Salad

Prep Time: 10 minutes **Cook Time:** 0 minutes
Servings: 1

Ingredients:
5 ounces canned sardines in oil
1 tablespoons lemon juice
1 small cucumber, chopped
½ tablespoon mustard
Salt and ground black pepper, to taste

Directions:
1.Drain sardines, put them in a bowl and mash using a fork.
2.Add salt, pepper, cucumber, lemon juice, and mustard, stir well, and serve cold.

Nutrition: Calories: 509, Fat: 32.5, Fiber: 1.6, Carbohydrates: 11.3, Protein: 42.1

Irish Clams

Prep Time: 10 minutes **Cook Time:** 10 minutes
Servings: 4

Ingredients:
2 pounds clams, scrubbed
3 ounces pancetta
1 tablespoon olive oil
3 tablespoons butter
2 garlic cloves, peeled and minced
1 bottle infused cider
Salt and ground black pepper, to taste
Juice of ½ lemon
2 thyme sprigs, chopped

Directions:
1.Heat a pan with oil over medium–high heat, add pancetta, brown for 3 minutes, reduce temperature to medium.
2.Add butter, garlic, salt, pepper, shallot, stir, and cook for 3 minutes.
3.Increase heat again, add cider, stir well, cook for 1 minute.
4.Add clams and thyme, cover pan, and simmer for 5 minutes.
5.Discard any unopened clams, add lemon juice, stir, divide into bowls. Serve hot.

Nutrition: Calories: 389, Fat: 21.5, Fiber: 1, Carbohydrates: 39.2, Protein: 9.5

Seared Scallops with Walnuts and Pomegranate

Prep Time: 5 minutes **Cook Time:** 10 minutes
Servings: 4

Ingredients:
1 pound scallops
3 tablespoons olive oil
1 shallot, peeled and chopped
3 garlic cloves, peeled and minced
2 cups spinach
1 cup chicken stock
1½ cups pomegranate seeds
¼ cup walnuts, toasted and chopped
1 tablespoon butter
Salt and ground black pepper, to taste

Directions:
1.Put romanesco in a food processor, blend, transfer to a bowl.
2.Heat a pan with 2 tablespoons oil over medium–high heat, add shallot and garlic, stir, and cook for 1 minute.
3.Add romanesco, spinach,1 cup stock, stir, cook for 3 minutes, blend using an immersion blender and take off the heat.
4.Heat another pan with 1 tablespoon oil and butter over medium–high heat, add scallops, season with salt and pepper, cook for 2 minutes, flip, and sear for 1 minute.
5.Divide romanesco mixture on plates, add scallops on side, top with walnuts and pomegranate, and serve.

Nutrition: Calories: 409, Fat: 19.1, Fiber: 2.2, Carbohydrates: 37.4, Protein: 23.3

Lemon–glazed Salmon

Prep Time: 10 minutes **Cook Time:** 10 minutes
Servings: 2

Ingredients:
2 lemons, sliced
1 pound wild salmon, skinless and cubed
¼ cup balsamic vinegar
¼ cup lemon juice
1 teaspoon coconut oil
⅓ cup no–sugar added lemon marmalade

Directions:
1.Heat a pot over medium heat, add vinegar, lemon juice, marmalade, stir well, bring to a simmer for 1 minute, reduce temperature, cook until it thickens a bit, and take off the heat.
2.Arrange salmon, lemon slices on skewers, and brush them on one side with the lemon glaze.
3.Brush a kitchen grill with coconut oil and heat over medium heat.
4.Place salmon kebabs on grill glazed side down and cook for 4 minutes.
5.Flip the kebabs, brush with the rest of the orange glaze, cook for 4 minutes, and serve.

Nutrition: Calories: 332, Fat: 13.3, Fiber: 2.5, Carbohydrates: 21.3, Protein: 34.1

Oysters with Pico De Gallo

Prep Time: 10 minutes **Cook Time:** 10 minutes
Servings: 6

Ingredients:
18 oysters, scrubbed
½ cup fresh cilantro, chopped
2 tomatoes, cored and chopped
1 jalapeño pepper, chopped
¼ cup onion, diced
Salt and ground black pepper, to taste
½ cup Monterey Jack cheese, shredded
2 limes, cut into wedges
Juice from 1 lime

Directions:
1.In a bowl, mix onion with jalapeño, cilantro, tomatoes, salt, pepper, lime juice, and stir well.
2.Place oysters on a preheated grill over medium–high heat, cover grill, and cook for 7 minutes until they open.
3.Transfer oysters to a heatproof dish, discarding any unopened ones.
4.Top oysters with cheese, and place under a preheated broiler for 1 minute.
5.Arrange oysters on a platter, top each with tomato 'Pico de Gallo' mixture and serve with lime wedges.

Nutrition: Calories: 174, Fat: 7.3, Fiber: 0.7, Carbohydrates: 9.1, Protein: 17.2

Grilled Squid with Guacamole

Prep Time: 10 minutes **Cook Time:** 10 minutes
Servings: 2

Ingredients:
2 medium squids, tentacles separated and tubes scored lengthwise
A drizzle of olive oil
Juice from 1 lime
Salt and ground black pepper, to taste
For the guacamole:
2 avocados, pitted, peeled, and chopped
Fresh coriander, chopped
2 red chilies, chopped
1 tomato, cored and chopped
1 onion, peeled and chopped
Juice from 2 limes

Directions:
1.Season squid and tentacles with salt, pepper, drizzle some olive oil, and massage well.
2.Place preheated grill pan over medium–high heat score side down, and cook for 2 minutes.
3.Flip and cook for 2 minutes, and transfer to a bowl.
4.Add juice from 1 lime, toss to coat, and keep warm.
5.Put avocado in a bowl and mash using a fork. Add coriander, chilies, tomato, onion, and juice from 2 limes, and stir.
6.Divide squid on plates, top with guacamole, and serve.

Nutrition: Calories: 779, Fat: 44.6, Fiber: 20.7, Carbohydrates: 47.9, Protein: 53.3

Mustard–glazed Salmon

Prep Time: 10 minutes **Cook Time:** 20 minutes
Servings: 1

Ingredients:
1 salmon fillet
Salt and ground black pepper, to taste
2 tablespoons mustard
1 tablespoon coconut oil
1 tablespoon sugar–free maple syrup

Directions:
1.In a bowl, mix sugar–free maple syrup with the mustard, and whisk.
2.Season salmon with salt and pepper, and brush the salmon with half of the mustard mixture.
3.Heat a pan with the oil over medium–high heat, place salmon flesh side down, and cook for 5 minutes.
4.Brush salmon with rest of the mustard mixture, transfer to a baking dish, place in an oven at 425ºF, bake for 15 minutes, and serve.

Nutrition: Calories: 465, Fat: 31, Fiber: 3.3, Carbohydrates: 9.6, Protein: 40.1

Shrimp and Cauliflower

Prep Time: 10 minutes **Cook Time:** 15 minutes
Servings: 2

Ingredients:
1 tablespoon butter
1 cauliflower head, separated into florets
1 pound shrimp, peeled and deveined
¼ cup coconut milk
8 ounces mushrooms, chopped
A pinch of red pepper flakes
Salt and ground black pepper, to taste
2 garlic cloves, peeled and minced
4 bacon slices
½ cup beef stock
1 tablespoon fresh parsley, diced
1 tablespoon fresh chives, chopped

Directions:
1.Heat a pan over medium–high heat, add bacon, cook until crispy, transfer to paper towels and leave aside.
2.Heat another pan with 1 tablespoon bacon fat over medium–high heat, add the shrimp, cook for 2 minutes on each side and transfer to a bowl.
3.Heat the pan again over medium heat, add mushrooms, stir, and cook for 3–4 minutes. Add garlic and pepper flakes, stir, and cook for 1 minute.
4.Add beef stock, salt, pepper, and return shrimp to pan. Stir, cook until everything thickens, take off heat and keep warm.
5.Meanwhile, put cauliflower in a food processor and mince it. Place into a heated pan over medium–high heat, stir, and cook for 5 minutes.
6.Add butter, stir, and blend using an immersion blender.
7.Add salt and pepper to taste, stir, divide into bowls.
8.Top with shrimp mixture, serve with parsley and chives.

Nutrition: Calories: 657, Fat: 33.1, Fiber: 5.2, Carbohydrates: 17.4, Protein: 72.9

Salmon with Arugula and Cabbage

Prep Time: 10 minutes **Cook Time:** 15 minutes
Servings: 4

Ingredients:
3 cups ice water
2 teaspoons sriracha sauce
3 scallions, chopped
Salt and ground black pepper, to taste
2 teaspoons flaxseed oil
4 teaspoons apple cider vinegar
4 medium salmon fillets
4 cups baby arugula
2 cups cabbage, shredded
1½ teaspoon Jamaican jerk seasoning
¼ cup sunflower seeds, toasted
2 cups watermelon radish, julienned

Directions:
1.Put ice water in a bowl, add scallions, and set aside. In another bowl, mix sriracha sauce with stevia and stir well.
2.Transfer 2 teaspoons of mixture to a bowl, and mix with half of the avocado oil, flaxseed oil, vinegar, salt, pepper, and whisk.
3.Sprinkle jerk seasoning over the salmon, rub with sriracha and stevia mixture, season with salt and pepper.
4.Heat a pan with rest of avocado oil over medium–high heat, add salmon, flesh side down, cook for 4 minutes, flip, and cook for 4 minutes, and divide on plates.
5.In a bowl, mix radishes with cabbage, and arugula.
6.Add salt, pepper, sriracha, and vinegar mixture, and toss well.
7.Add to salmon fillets, drizzle the remaining sriracha, and stevia sauce all over and top with sunflower seeds and drained scallions.

Nutrition: Calories: 417, Fat: 21.5, Fiber: 4.2, Carbohydrates: 20.2, Protein: 39.3

Scallops with Fennel Sauce

Prep Time: 10 minutes **Cook Time:** 10 minutes
Servings: 2

Ingredients:
6 scallops
1 fennel bulb, trimmed, leaves chopped, and cut into wedges
Juice of ½ lime
1 lime, cut into wedges
Zest from 1 lime
1 egg yolk
3 tablespoons butter, melted, and heated up
½ tablespoons olive oil
Salt and ground black pepper, to taste

Directions:
1.Season scallops with salt, and pepper, put in a bowl, and mix with half of the lime juice, and half of the zest, and toss to coat.
2.In a bowl, mix egg yolk with some salt and pepper and rest of lime juice and lime zest, and whisk.
3.Add melted butter and fennel wedges and stir.
4.Brush fennel wedges with oil, place on heated grill pan over medium–high heat, cook for 2 minutes, flip, and cook for 2 minutes.
5.Add scallops on grill, cook for 2 minutes, flip, and cook for 2 minutes.
6.Divide fennel and scallops on plates, drizzle fennel and butter mixture, and serve with lime wedges on the side.

Nutrition: Calories: 335, Fat: 24, Fiber: 4.6, Carbohydrates: 14.5, Protein: 18.3

Salmon with Lemon Relish

Prep Time: 10 minutes **Cook Time:** 1 hour
Servings: 2

Ingredients:
2 medium salmon fillets
Salt and ground black pepper, to taste
A drizzle of olive oil
1 shallot, peeled and chopped
1 tablespoon lemon juice
1 lemon
¼ cup olive oil
2 tablespoons fresh parsley, diced

Directions:
1.Brush salmon fillets with a drizzle of olive oil, sprinkle with salt and pepper, place on a lined baking sheet, place in an oven at 400ºF, and bake for 1 hour.
2.Meanwhile, put shallot in a bowl, add 1 tablespoon lemon juice, salt, and pepper, stir, and set aside for 10 minutes.
3.Cut lemon into thin wedges.
4.Add to shallots with the parsley and ¼ cup olive oil and stir.
5.Take salmon out of the oven, break into medium pieces, and serve with the lemon relish on the side.

Nutrition: Calories: 548, Fat: 43.4, Fiber: 1, Carbohydrates: 9, Protein: 35.9

Mussel Soup

Prep Time: 10 minutes **Cook Time:** 15 minutes
Servings: 6

Ingredients:
2 pounds mussels
28 ounces canned crushed tomatoes
28 ounces canned diced tomatoes
2 cup chicken stock
1 teaspoon red pepper flakes
3 garlic cloves, peeled and minced
½ cup fresh parsley, chopped
1 onion, peeled and chopped
Salt and ground black pepper, to taste
1 tablespoon olive oil

Directions:
1.Heat up a Dutch oven with oil over medium–high heat, add onion, stir, and cook for 3 minutes.
2.Add garlic and red pepper flakes, stir, and cook for 1 minute.
3.Add tomatoes and stir. Add chicken stock, salt, pepper, stir, and bring to a boil.
4.Add rinsed mussels, salt, pepper, cook until they open, discard any unopened ones and mix with parsley.
5.Stir, divide into bowls, and serve.

Nutrition: Calories: 242, Fat: 6.3, Fiber: 6.5, Carbohydrates: 24.3, Protein: 23.1

Fish Pie

Prep Time: 10 minutes **Cook Time:** 1 hour and 10 minutes
Servings: 6

Ingredients:
1 onion, peeled and chopped
2 salmon fillets, skinless and cut into medium–sized pieces
2 mackerel fillets, skinless and cut into medium–sized pieces
3 haddock fillets, cut into medium–sized pieces
¼ cup butter+ 2 tablespoons butter
1 cauliflower head, separated into florets
4 eggs
4 cloves
1 cup whipping cream
½ cup water
A pinch of nutmeg, ground
1 teaspoon Dijon mustard
1 cup cheddar cheese, shredded+ ½ cup cheddar cheese, shredded
Some chopped parsley
Salt and ground black pepper, to taste
4 tablespoons fresh chives, chopped

Directions:
1.Put some water in a saucepan, add some salt, bring to a boil over medium heat, add eggs, cook them for 10 minutes, take off the heat, drain, leave them to cool down, peel, and cut them into quarters.
2.Put the water in another saucepan, bring to a boil, add the cauliflower florets, cook for 10 minutes, drain them, transfer to a blender, add the ¼ cup butter, pulse well, and transfer to a bowl.
3.Put the cream and ½ cup water in a pan, add the fish, toss to coat, and heat over medium heat.
4.Add onion, cloves, bring to a boil, reduce heat, and simmer for 10 minutes.
5.Take off heat, transfer fish to a baking dish, and set aside. Return the pan with fish sauce to heat, add the nutmeg, stir, and cook for 5 minutes.
6.Take off heat, discard the cloves and bay leaves, add 1 cup cheddar cheese, 2 tablespoons butter, and stir well.
7.Place egg quarters on top of the fish in the baking dish.
8.Add cream and cheese sauce over them, top with cauliflower mash, sprinkle rest of the cheddar cheese, chives, parsley, place in an oven at 400ºF for 30 minutes.
9.Let the pie to cool before slicing, and serving.

Nutrition: Calories: 120, Fat: 8.4, Fiber: 3.1, Carbohydrates: 8.1, Protein: 5

Salmon Stuffed with Shrimp

Prep Time: 10 minutes **Cook Time:** 25 minutes
Servings: 2

Ingredients:
2 salmon fillets
A drizzle of olive oil
5 ounces tiger shrimp, peeled, deveined, and chopped
6 mushrooms, chopped
3 green onions, chopped
2 cups spinach
¼ cup macadamia nuts, toasted and chopped
Salt and ground black pepper, to taste
A pinch of nutmeg
¼ cup mayonnaise

Directions:
1.Heat a pan with the oil over medium–high heat, add mushrooms, onions, salt, and pepper, stir, and cook for 4 minutes.
2.Add macadamia nuts, stir, and cook for 2 minutes. Add spinach, stir, and cook for 1 minute. Add shrimp, stir, and cook for 1 minute.
3.Take off heat, set aside for a few minutes, add mayonnaise, nutmeg, and stir well.
4.Make an incision lengthwise in each salmon fillet, sprinkle salt, and pepper, divide spinach and shrimp mixture into incisions, and place on a working surface.
5.Heat a pan with a drizzle of oil over medium–high heat, add stuffed salmon, skin side down, cook for 1 minutes, reduce temperature, cover pan, and cook for 8 minutes.
6.Broil for 3 minutes, divide on plates, and serve.

Nutrition: Calories: 567, Fat: 34.6, Fiber: 3.3, Carbohydrates: 13.9, Protein: 53.9

Baked Haddock

Prep Time: 10 minutes **Cook Time:** 30 minutes
Servings: 4

Ingredients:
1 pound haddock
3 teaspoons water
2 tablespoons lemon juice
Salt and ground black pepper, to taste
2 tablespoons mayonnaise
1 teaspoon dill weed
Vegetable oil cooking spray
A pinch of Old Bay Seasoning

Directions:
1.Spray a baking dish with some cooking oil.
2.Add lemon juice, water, fish, and toss to coat. Add salt, pepper, Old Bay Seasoning, dill, and toss again. Add mayonnaise and spread well.
3.Place in an oven at 350ºF, and bake for 30 minutes. Divide on plates and serve.

Nutrition: Calories: 121, Fat: 3.5, Fiber: 0, Carbohydrates: 1.9, Protein:20.1

Tilapia

Prep Time: 10 minutes **Cook Time:** 10 minutes
Servings: 4

Ingredients:
4 tilapia fillets, boneless
Salt and ground black pepper, to taste
½ cup Parmesan cheese, grated
4 tablespoons mayonnaise
¼ teaspoon dried basil
¼ teaspoon garlic powder
2 tablespoons lemon juice
¼ cup butter
Vegetable oil cooking spray
A pinch of onion powder

Directions:
1.Spray a baking sheet with cooking spray, and arrange the tilapia on the tray.
2.Season with salt, pepper, place under a preheated broiler, and cook for 3 minutes.
3.Turn the fish and broil for 3 minutes.
4.In a bowl, mix Parmesan cheese with mayonnaise, basil, garlic, lemon juice, onion powder, butter, and stir well.
5.Add fish to mixture, toss to coat well, place on baking sheet again, and broil for 3 minutes. Transfer to plates and serve.

Nutrition: Calories: 300, Fat: 20.5, Fiber: 0.1, Carbohydrates: 4.3, Protein: 25.9

Salmon with Caper Sauce

Prep Time: 10 minutes **Cook Time:** 20 minutes
Servings: 3

Ingredients:
3 salmon fillets
Salt and ground black pepper, to taste
1 tablespoon olive oil
1 tablespoon Italian seasoning
2 tablespoons capers
3 tablespoons lemon juice
4 garlic cloves, peeled and minced
2 tablespoons butter

Directions:
1.Heat a pan with olive oil over medium heat, add fish fillets skin side up, season with salt, pepper, and Italian seasoning, cook for 2 minutes, flip, and cook for 2 minutes, take off heat, cover pan, and set aside for 15 minutes.
2.Transfer fish to a plate, and leave them aside.
3.Heat the same pan over medium heat, add capers, lemon juice, and garlic, stir, and cook for 2 minutes.
4.Take pan off the heat, add the butter, and stir well.
5.Return fish to pan, and toss to coat with the sauce. Divide on plates and serve.

Nutrition: Calories: 369, Fat: 24.9, Fiber: 0.3, Carbohydrates: 2.4, Protein: 35.

Trout with Butter Sauce

Prep Time: 10 minutes **Cook Time:** 10 minutes
Servings: 4

Ingredients:
4 trout fillets
Salt and ground black pepper, to taste
3 teaspoons lemon zest, grated
3 tablespoons fresh chives, chopped
6 tablespoons butter
2 tablespoons olive oil
2 teaspoons lemon juice

Directions:
1.Season trout with salt, pepper, drizzle olive oil, and massage into fish.
2.Heat a kitchen grill over medium–high heat, add fish fillets, cook for 4 minutes, flip, and cook for 4 minutes.
3.Heat a pan with the butter over medium heat, add salt, pepper, chives, lemon juice, lemon zest, and stir well.
4.Divide fish fillets on plates, drizzle the butter sauce over them, and serve.

Nutrition: Calories: 333, Fat: 29.6, Fiber: 0.2, Carbohydrates: 0.5, Protein: 16.8

Roasted Salmon

Prep Time: 10 minutes **Cook Time:** 12 minutes
Servings: 4

Ingredients:
2 tablespoons butter, softened
1¼ pound salmon fillet
2 ounces kimchi, diced
Salt and ground black pepper, to taste

Directions:
1.In a food processor, mix butter with kimchi and blend well.
2.Rub salmon with salt, pepper, and kimchi mixture, and place into a baking dish.
3.Place in an oven at 425ºF and bake for 15 minutes. Divide on plates and serve.

Nutrition: Calories: 467, Fat: 25, Fiber: 0, Carbohydrates: 0.5, Protein: 60.6

Salmon Meatballs

Prep Time: 10 minutes **Cook Time:** 30 minutes
Servings: 4

Ingredients:
2 tablespoons butter
2 garlic cloves, peeled and minced
⅓ cup onion, peeled and chopped
1 pound wild salmon, boneless and minced
¼ cup fresh chives, chopped
1 egg
2 tablespoons Dijon mustard
1 tablespoon coconut flour
Salt and ground black pepper, to taste
For the sauce:
4 garlic cloves, peeled and minced
2 tablespoons butter
2 tablespoons Dijon mustard
Juice, and zest of 1 lemon
2 cups coconut cream
2 tablespoons fresh chives, chopped

Directions:
1.Heat a pan with 2 tablespoons butter over medium heat, add onion and 2 garlic cloves, stir, cook for 3 minutes, and transfer to a bowl.
2.In another bowl, mix the onion and garlic with salmon, chives, coconut flour, salt, pepper, 2 tablespoons mustard, egg, and stir well.
3.Shape meatballs from salmon mixture, place on a baking sheet, place in an oven at 350ºF, and bake for 25 minutes.
4.Heat a pan with 2 tablespoons butter over medium heat, add 4 garlic cloves, stir, and cook for 1 minute.
5.Add coconut cream, 2 tablespoons Dijon mustard, lemon juice, lemon zest, chives, stir, and cook for 3 minutes.
6.Take salmon meatballs out of the oven, drop them into the Dijon sauce, toss, cook for 1 minute, and take off the heat. Divide into bowls and serve.

Nutrition: Calories: 575, Fat: 47.1, Fiber: 3.4, Carbohydrates: 9, Protein: 31.9

Simple Grilled Oysters

Prep Time: 10 minutes **Cook Time:** 10 minutes
Servings: 3

Ingredients:
6 oysters, shucked
3 garlic cloves, peeled and minced
1 lemon, cut in wedges
1 tablespoon parsley
A pinch of sweet paprika
2 tablespoons melted butter

Directions:
1.Top each oyster with melted butter, parsley, paprika, and butter.
2.Place on preheated grill pan over medium–high heat, and cook for 8 minutes.
3.Serve them with lemon wedges on the side.

Nutrition: Calories: 272, Fat: 15.7, Fiber: 0.1, Carbohydrates: 13, Protein: 20.3

Trout with Special Sauce

Prep Time: 10 minutes **Cook Time:** 10 minutes
Servings: 1

Ingredients:
1 trout fillet
Salt and ground black pepper, to taste
1 tablespoon olive oil
1 tablespoon butter
Zest, and juice from 1 lemon
½ cup fresh parsley, chopped
½ cup pecans, chopped

Directions:
1.Heat a pan with the oil over medium–high heat, add fish fillet, season with salt, pepper, cook for 4 minutes on each side, transfer to a plate and keep warm.
2.Heat the same pan with butter over medium heat, add pecans, stir, and toast for 1 minutes.
3.Add lemon juice, lemon zest, some salt, pepper, and chopped parsley, stir, cook for 1 minute, and pour over the fish fillets, and serve.

Nutrition: Calories: 838, Fat: 81, Fiber: 8.5, Carbohydrates: 11.9, Protein: 25

Crusted Salmon

Prep Time: 10 minutes **Cook Time:** 15 minutes
Servings: 4

Ingredients:
3 garlic cloves, peeled and minced
2 pounds salmon fillet
Salt and ground black pepper, to taste
½ cup Parmesan cheese, grated
¼ cup fresh parsley, chopped

Directions:
1.Place salmon on a lined baking sheet, season with salt, and pepper, cover with a parchment paper, place in an oven at 425ºF, and bake for 10 minutes.
2.Take fish out of the oven, sprinkle Parmesan cheese, parsley, and garlic over fish, place in an oven again, and cook for 5 minutes.
3.Divide on plates and serve.

Nutrition: Calories: 350, Fat: 17, Fiber: 1.5, Carbohydrates: 0.2, Protein: 48.8

Sour Cream Salmon

Prep Time: 10 minutes **Cook Time:** 15 minutes
Servings: 4

Ingredients:
4 salmon fillets
A drizzle of olive oil
Salt and ground black pepper, to taste
⅓ cup Parmesan cheese, grated
1½ teaspoon mustard
½ cup sour cream

Directions:
1.Place salmon on a lined baking sheet, season with salt, and pepper, and drizzle the oil. In a bowl, mix sour cream with Parmesan cheese, mustard, salt, pepper, and stir well.
2.Spoon sour cream mixture over the salmon, place in an oven at 350ºF, and bake for 15 minutes. Divide on plates and serve.

Nutrition: Calories: 319, Fat: 18.5, Fiber: 0, Carbohydrates: 1.5, Protein: 37.7

Grilled Salmon

Prep Time: 30 minutes **Cook Time:** 10 minutes
Servings: 4

Ingredients:
4 salmon fillets
1 tablespoon olive oil
Salt and ground black pepper, to taste
1 teaspoon cumin
1 teaspoon sweet paprika
½ teaspoon chili powder
1 teaspoon onion powder
For the salsa:
1 onion, peeled and chopped
1 avocado, pitted, peeled, and chopped
2 tablespoons fresh cilantro, chopped
Juice from 2 limes
Salt and ground black pepper, to taste

Directions:
1.In a bowl, mix salt, pepper, chili powder, onion powder, paprika, and cumin.
2.Rub salmon with this mixture, drizzle the oil, rub again, and cook on preheated grill pan for 4 minutes on each side.
3.In a bowl, mix avocado with onion, salt, pepper, cilantro, lime juice, and stir.
4.Divide salmon on plates and top each fillet with avocado salsa.

Nutrition: Calories: 379, Fat: 24.3, Fiber: 4, Carbohydrates: 6.9, Protein: 35.8

Tuna Cakes

Prep Time: 10 minutes **Cook Time:** 10 minutes
Servings: 12

Ingredients:
15 ounces canned tuna, drained well and flaked
3 eggs
½ teaspoon dried dill
1 teaspoon dried parsley
½ cup onion chopped
1 teaspoon garlic powder
Salt and ground black pepper, to taste
Oil, for frying

Directions:
1.In a bowl, mix tuna with salt, pepper, dill, parsley, onion, garlic powder, eggs, and stir well.
2.Shape tuna cakes and place on a plate.
3.Heat a pan with oil over medium–high heat, add tuna cakes, cook for 5 minutes on each side. Divide on plates and serve.

Nutrition: Calories: 84, Fat: 4, Fiber: 0.1, Carbohydrates: 0.6, Protein: 10.8

Baked Halibut

Prep Time: 10 minutes **Cook Time:** 10 minutes
Servings: 4

Ingredients:
½ cup Parmesan cheese, grated
¼ cup butter
¼ cup mayonnaise
2 tablespoons green onions, chopped
6 garlic cloves, peeled and minced
A dash of Tabasco sauce
4 halibut fillets
Salt and ground black pepper, to taste
Juice of ½ lemon

Directions:
1.Season halibut with salt, pepper, and some of the lemon juice, place in a baking dish, and cook in the oven at 450ºF for 6 minutes.
2.Heat a pan with butter over medium heat, add Parmesan cheese, mayonnaise, green onions, Tabasco sauce, garlic, remaining lemon juice, and stir well.
3.Take fish out of the oven, drizzle cheese sauce all over, turn the oven to broil, and broil the fish for 3 minutes. Divide on plates and serve.

Nutrition: Calories: 530, Fat: 26.2, Fiber: 0.2, Carbohydrates: 5.7, Protein: 65.6

Pan–roasted Cod

Prep Time: 10 minutes **Cook Time:** 20 minutes
Servings: 4

Ingredients:
1 pound cod, cut into medium–sized pieces
Salt and ground black pepper, to taste
2 green onions, chopped
3 garlic cloves, peeled and minced
3 tablespoons soy sauce
1 cup fish stock
1 tablespoon balsamic vinegar
1 tablespoon fresh ginger, grated
½ teaspoon red chili flakes

Directions:
1.Heat a pan over medium–high heat, add fish pieces, and brown on each side.
2.Add garlic, green onions, salt, pepper, soy sauce, fish stock, vinegar, chili pepper, ginger, stir, cover, reduce heat, and cook for 20 minutes.
3.Divide on plates and serve.

Nutrition: Calories: 131, Fat: 1, Fiber: 0.4, Carbohydrates: 2.2, Protein: 26.9

Sea Bass with Capers

Prep Time: 10 minutes **Cook Time:** 15 minutes
Servings: 4

Ingredients:
1 lemon, sliced
1 pound sea bass fillet
2 tablespoons capers
2 tablespoons fresh dill
Salt and ground black pepper, to taste

Directions:
1.Put sea bass fillet into a baking dish, season with salt, and pepper, add capers, dill, and lemon slices on top.
2.Place in an oven at 350ºF and bake for 15 minutes. Divide on plates and serve.

Nutrition: Calories: 150, Fat: 3.1, Fiber: 0.8, Carbohydrates: 2.4, Protein: 27.4

Cod with Arugula

Prep Time: 10 minutes **Cook Time:** 20 minutes
Servings: 2

Ingredients:
2 cod fillets
1 tablespoon olive oil
Salt and ground black pepper, to taste
Juice of 1 lemon
3 cup arugula
½ cup black olives, pitted and sliced
2 tablespoons capers
1 garlic clove, peeled and chopped

Directions:
1.Arrange fish fillets in a heatproof dish, season with salt, pepper, drizzle the oil and lemon juice, toss to coat, place in an oven at 450ºF, and bake for 20 minutes.
2.In a food processor, mix arugula with salt, pepper, capers, olives, garlic, and blend well.
3.Arrange the fish on plates, top with arugula tapenade, and serve.

Nutrition: Calories: 294, Fat: 12.9, Fiber: 2.3, Carbohydrates: 5.8, Protein: 41.4

Sautéed Lemon Shrimp

Prep Time: 10 minutes **Cook Time:** 10 minutes
Servings: 4

Ingredients:
2 tablespoons olive oil
1 tablespoon butter
1 pound shrimp, peeled and deveined
2 tablespoons lemon juice
2 tablespoons garlic, minced
1 tablespoon lemon zest
Salt and ground black pepper, to taste

Directions:
1.Heat a pan with oil and butter over medium–high heat, add shrimp, and cook for 2 minutes.
2.Add garlic, stir, and cook for 4 minutes.
3.Add lemon juice, lemon zest, salt, and pepper, stir, take off the heat, and serve.

Nutrition: Calories: 220, Fat: 11.8, Fiber: 0.1, Carbohydrates: 1.7, Protein: 25.9

Baked Halibut with Vegetables

Prep Time: 10 minutes **Cook Time:** 35 minutes
Servings: 2

Ingredients:
1 red bell pepper, seeded and chopped
1 yellow bell pepper, seeded and chopped
1 teaspoon balsamic vinegar
1 tablespoon olive oil
2 halibut fillets
2 cups baby spinach
Salt and ground black pepper, to taste
1 teaspoon cumin

Directions:
1.In a bowl, mix bell peppers with salt, pepper, half of the oil, and vinegar, toss to coat well, and transfer to a baking dish.
2.Place in oven at 400ºF, and bake for 20 minutes.
3.Heat a pan with the rest of the oil over medium heat, add fish, season with salt, pepper, cumin, and brown on all sides.
4.Take baking dish out of the oven, add the spinach, stir gently, and divide the whole mixture on plates.
5.Add fish on the side, sprinkle with salt and pepper, and serve.

Nutrition: Calories: 404, Fat: 14, Fiber: 1.5, Carbohydrates: 5.6, Protein: 62

Roasted Sea Bass

Prep Time: 10 minutes **Cook Time:** 12 minutes
Servings: 4

Ingredients:
2 sea bass fillets
2 teaspoon olive oil
2 teaspoons Italian seasoning
¼ cup green olives, pitted and chopped
¼ cup cherry tomatoes, cored and chopped
¼ cup black olives, chopped
1 tablespoon lemon zest
2 tablespoons lemon zest
Salt and ground black pepper, to taste
2 tablespoons fresh parsley, chopped
1 tablespoon olive oil

Directions:
1.Rub fish with salt, pepper, Italian seasoning, and 2 teaspoons olive oil, transfer to a baking dish and set aside.
2.In a bowl, mix tomatoes with all the olives, salt, pepper, lemon zest, and lemon juice, parsley, 1 tablespoon olive oil, and toss well.
3.Place fish in the oven at 400ºF, and bake for 12 minutes.
4.Divide fish on plates, top with tomato relish, and serve.

Nutrition: Calories: 133, Fat: 7.8, Fiber: 1.4, Carbohydrates: 3.5, Protein: 12.5

Coconut Shrimp

Prep Time: 10 minutes **Cook Time:** 13 minutes
Servings: 4

Ingredients:
1 pound shrimp, peeled and deveined
Salt and ground black pepper, to taste
4 cherry tomatoes, cored and chopped
1 red bell pepper, seeded and sliced
1 tablespoon olive oil
½ cup fresh cilantro, chopped
1 tablespoon garlic, minced
½ cup green onion, peeled and chopped
½ teaspoon red pepper flakes
10 ounces coconut milk
2 tablespoons lime juice

Directions:
1.Heat a pan with oil over medium–high heat, add pepper and cook for 3 minutes.
2.Add cilantro, garlic, green onions, and pepper flakes, stir, and cook for 1 minute.
3.Add tomatoes, and coconut milk, stir, and simmer everything for 5 minutes.
4.Add shrimp and lime juice, stir, and cook for 3 minutes.
5.Season with salt and pepper, stir, and serve hot.

Nutrition: Calories: 368, Fat: 22.7, Fiber: 3.9, Carbohydrates: 14.7, Protein: 29.3

Shrimp and Noodle Salad

Prep Time: 10 minutes **Cook Time:** 0 minutes
Servings: 4

Ingredients:
1 cucumber, cut with a spiralizer
½ cup fresh basil, chopped
½ pound shrimp, already cooked, peeled and deveined
Salt and ground black pepper, to taste
1 tablespoon stevia
2 teaspoons fish sauce
2 tablespoons lime juice
2 teaspoons tomato paste
½ teaspoons chili powder

Directions:
1.Put cucumber noodles on a paper towel, cover with another one, and press well.
2.Put into a bowl and mix with basil, shrimp, salt, and pepper.
3.In another bowl, mix stevia with fish sauce, lime juice, chili powder and tomato paste, and whisk.
4.Add to the shrimp salad, toss to coat well, and serve.

Nutrition: Calories: 84, Fat: 1.1, Fiber: 0.6, Carbohydrates: 5.2, Protein: 13.8

Roasted Mahi Mahi and Tomato

Prep Time: 10 minutes **Cook Time:** 16 minutes
Servings: 2

Ingredients:
2 mahi mahi fillets
½ cup onion, peeled and chopped
4 teaspoons olive oil
1 teaspoon Greek seasoning
1 teaspoon garlic, minced
1 green bell pepper, seeded and chopped
½ cup tomato passata
2 tablespoons Kalamata olives, pitted and chopped
¼ cup chicken stock
Salt and ground black pepper, to taste
2 tablespoons feta cheese, crumbled

Directions:
1.Heat a pan with 2 teaspoons oil over medium heat, add bell pepper and onion, stir, and cook for 3 minutes.
2.Add Greek seasoning and garlic, stir, and cook for 1 minute.
3.Add stock, olives, and tomato passata, stir again, and cook for 5 minutes or until mixture thickens. Transfer to a bowl and set aside.
4.Heat the pan again with rest of the oil over medium heat, add the fish, season with salt and pepper, and cook for 2 minutes.
5.Flip, cook for 2 minutes, and transfer to a baking dish.
6.Spoon salsa over fish, place in an oven, and bake at 425ºF for 6 minutes. Sprinkle feta on top and serve hot.

Nutrition: Calories: 368, Fat: 14.4, Fiber: 1.7, Carbohydrates: 17.6, Protein: 42.2

Spicy Shrimp

Prep Time: 10 minutes **Cook Time:** 8 minutes
Servings: 2

Ingredients:
½ pound shrimp, peeled and deveined
2 teaspoons Worcestershire sauce
2 teaspoons olive oil
Juice of 1 lemon
Salt and ground black pepper, to taste
1 teaspoon Creole seasoning

Directions:
1.Arrange shrimp in one layer in a baking dish, season with salt, pepper, and drizzle the oil.
2.Add Worcestershire sauce, lemon juice, and sprinkle Creole seasoning.
3.Toss shrimp in the seasoning, place in an oven, set it under the broiler, and broil for 8 minutes.
4.Divide between 2 plates and serve.

Nutrition: Calories: 192, Fat: 6.7, Fiber: 1.2, Carbohydrates: 6.6, Protein: 26.3

Fish Curry

Prep Time: 10 minutes **Cook Time:** 25 minutes
Servings: 4

Ingredients:
4 white fish fillets
½ teaspoon mustard seeds
Salt and ground black pepper, to taste
2 green chilies, chopped
1 teaspoon fresh ginger, grated
1 teaspoon curry powder
¼ teaspoon cumin
4 tablespoons coconut oil
1 onion, peeled and chopped
1–inch turmeric root, grated
¼ cup fresh cilantro
1½ cups coconut cream
3 garlic cloves, peeled and minced

Directions:
1.Heat a saucepan with half of the coconut oil over medium heat, add mustard seeds, and cook for 2 minutes.
2.Add ginger, onion, garlic, stir, and cook for 5 minutes. Add turmeric, curry powder, chilies, and cumin, stir, and cook for 5 minutes.
3.Add coconut milk, salt, and pepper, stir, bring to a boil, and cook for 15 minutes.
4.Heat another pan with remaining oil over medium heat, add fish, stir, and cook for 3 minutes.
5.Add to curry sauce, stir, and cook for 5 minutes.
6.Add cilantro, stir, divide into bowls, and serve.

Nutrition: Calories: 1541, Fat: 138.5, Fiber: 10.6, Carbohydrates: 28.8, Protein: 60.9

Shrimp Stew

Prep Time: 10 minutes **Cook Time:** 15 minutes
Servings: 6

Ingredients:
¼ cup onion, peeled and chopped
¼ cup olive oil
1 garlic clove, peeled and minced
1½ pounds shrimp, peeled and deveined
¼ cup red pepper, roasted and chopped
14 ounces canned diced tomatoes
¼ cup fresh cilantro, chopped
2 tablespoons sriracha sauce
1 cup coconut milk
Salt and ground black pepper, to taste
2 tablespoons lime juice

Directions:
1.Heat a pan with oil over medium heat, add onion, stir, and cook for 4 minutes.
2.Add peppers and garlic, stir, and cook for 4 minutes.
3.Add cilantro, tomatoes, shrimp, stir, and cook until shrimp turns pink.
4.Add coconut milk and sriracha sauce, stir, and bring to a gentle simmer.
5.Add the salt, pepper, lime juice, stir, transfer to bowls, and serve.

Nutrition: Calories: 676, Fat: 25.1, Fiber: 1.9, Carbohydrates: 12.5, Protein: 96.3

Garlicky Mussels

Prep Time: 5 minutes **Cook Time:** 5 minutes
Servings: 4

Ingredients:
2 pound mussels, debearded and scrubbed
2 garlic cloves, peeled and minced
1 tablespoon butter
A splash of lemon juice

Directions:
1.Put some water in a saucepan, add mussels, bring to a boil over medium heat, cook for 5 minutes, take off heat, discard any unopened mussels, and transfer them to a bowl.
2.In another bowl, mix butter with garlic and lemon juice, whisk, and heat in the microwave for 1 minute.
3.Pour over mussels and serve.

Nutrition: Calories: 224, Fat: 8, Fiber: 0.1, Carbohydrates: 9, Protein: 27.2

Shrimp Alfredo

Prep Time: 10 minutes **Cook Time:** 20 minutes
Servings: 4

Ingredients:
8 ounces mushrooms, chopped
1 asparagus bunch, cut into medium–sized pieces
1 pound shrimp, peeled and deveined
Salt and ground black pepper, to taste
1 spaghetti squash, cut in half
2 tablespoons olive oil
2 teaspoons Italian seasoning
1 onion, peeled and chopped
1 teaspoon red pepper flakes
¼ cup butter
1 cup Parmesan cheese, grated
2 garlic cloves, peeled and minced
1 cup heavy cream

Directions:
1.Place squash halves on a lined baking sheet, place in an oven at 425ºF, and roast for 40 minutes.
2.Scoop out flesh and put into a bowl.
3.Put water in a saucepan, add some salt, bring to a boil over medium heat, add the asparagus, steam for a couple of minutes, transfer to a bowl filled with ice water, drain, and set aside.
4.Heat a pan with oil over medium heat, add onions and mushrooms, stir, and cook for 7 minutes.
5.Add pepper flakes, Italian seasoning, salt, pepper, squash, asparagus, stir, and cook for a few minutes.
6.Heat another pan with the butter over medium heat, add heavy cream, garlic, and Parmesan cheese, stir, and cook for 5 minutes.
7.Add shrimp to the pan, stir, and cook for 7 minutes.
8.Divide vegetables on plates, top with shrimp and sauce, and serve.

Nutrition: Calories: 531, Fat: 37.5, Fiber: 1.9, Carbohydrates: 15.2, Protein:36.7

Salmon Skewers

Prep Time: 10 minutes **Cook Time:** 8 minutes
Servings: 4

Ingredients:
12 ounces salmon fillet, cubed
1 onion, peeled and cut into chunks
½ red bell pepper, seeded and cut in chunks
½ green bell pepper, seeded and cut in chunks
½ orange bell pepper, seeded and cut in chunks
Juice from 1 lemon
Salt and ground black pepper, to taste
A drizzle of olive oil

Directions:
1.Thread skewers with onion, bell peppers, and salmon cubes.
2.Season with salt and pepper, drizzle them with oil and lemon juice, and place them on preheated grill over medium–high heat.
3.Cook for 4 minutes on each side, divide on plates, and serve.

Nutrition: Calories: 162, Fat: 5.6, Fiber: 2.2, Carbohydrates: 11.6, Protein: 18

Octopus Salad

Prep Time: 10 minutes **Cook Time:** 40 minutes
Servings: 2

Ingredients:
21 ounces octopus, rinsed
Juice of 1 lemon
4 celery stalks, chopped
3 ounces olive oil
Salt and ground black pepper, to taste
4 tablespoons fresh parsley, chopped

Directions:
1.Put octopus in a pot, add enough water to cover, place a lid on the pot, bring to a boil over medium heat, cook for 40 minutes, drain, and set aside to cool down.
2.Chop octopus and put it in a salad bowl.
3.Add celery stalks, parsley, oil, lemon juice, and toss well. Season with salt and pepper, toss again, and serve.

Nutrition: Calories: 839, Fat: 46, Fiber: 1.1, Carbohydrates: 15.6, Protein: 89.3

Shrimp and Tomato Soup

Prep Time: 10 minutes **Cook Time:** 10 minutes
Servings: 4

Ingredients:
4 scallions, chopped
1½ tablespoons coconut oil
1 small ginger root, diced
8 cups chicken stock
¼ cup coconut aminos
5 ounces canned bamboo shoots, drained and sliced
Ground black pepper, to taste
¼ teaspoon fish sauce
1 pound shrimp, peeled and deveined
½ pound tomatoes
1 tablespoon sesame oil
½ tablespoon chili oil

Directions:
1.Heat a pot with coconut oil over medium heat, add scallions and ginger, stir, and cook for 2 minutes.
2.Add coconut aminos, stock, black pepper, fish sauce, stir, and bring to a boil.
3.Add shrimp, chopped tomatoes, bamboo shoots, stir, and cook for 3 minutes.
4.Add sesame oil and hot chili oil, stir, divide into bowls, and serve.

Nutrition: Calories: 846, Fat: 26, Fiber: 1.9, Carbohydrates: 102.9, Protein: 27.5

Fried Calamari with Spicy Sauce

Prep Time: 10 minutes **Cook Time:** 20 minutes
Servings: 2

Ingredients:
1 squid, cut into medium rings
A pinch of cayenne pepper
1 egg, whisked
2 tablespoons coconut flour
Salt and ground black pepper, to taste
Coconut oil for frying
1 tablespoons lemon juice
4 tablespoons mayonnaise
1 teaspoon sriracha sauce

Directions:
1.Season squid rings with salt, pepper, and cayenne pepper, and put them in a bowl.
2.In another bowl, mix egg with salt, pepper, coconut flour, and whisk. Coat the calamari rings in the egg mixture.
3.Heat a pan with enough coconut oil over medium heat, add calamari rings, and cook them until they become golden brown on both sides.
4.Transfer to paper towels, drain excess grease, and put in a bowl.
5.In another bowl, mix mayonnaise with lemon juice and sriracha sauce, stir well, and serve the calamari rings with this sauce on the side.

Nutrition: Calories: 620, Fat: 42.9, Fiber: 0.3, Carbohydrates: 15.7, Protein: 42.9

Clam Chowder

Prep Time: 10 minutes **Cook Time:** 2 hours
Servings: 4

Ingredients:
1 cup celery stalks, chopped
Salt and ground black pepper, to taste
1 teaspoon ground thyme
2 cups chicken stock
14 ounces canned baby clams
2 cups heavy cream
1 cup onion, peeled and chopped
12 bacon slices, chopped

Directions:
1.Heat a pan over medium heat, add bacon slices, brown all over, transfer bacon to a bowl, reserving the bacon grease in the pan.
2.Heat the pan again, add celery onion, stir, and cook for 5 minutes.
3.Transfer everything including the bacon to a slow cooker with the baby clams, salt, pepper, stock, thyme, cream, stir, and cook on high for 2 hours.
4.Divide into bowls and serve.

Nutrition: Calories: 583, Fat: 46.6, Fiber: 1.4, Carbohydrates: 17.2, Protein: 23.8

Flounder and Shrimp

Prep Time: 10 minutes **Cook Time:** 20 minutes
Servings: 4

Ingredients:
For the seasoning:
½ teaspoon allspice
1 teaspoon dried oregano
¼ teaspoon ground nutmeg
¼ teaspoon ground cloves
A pinch of ground cinnamon
For the etouffee:
2 shallots, peeled and chopped
1 tablespoon butter
8 ounces bacon, sliced
1 green bell pepper, seeded and chopped
1 celery stalk, chopped
2 tablespoons coconut flour
1 tomato, cored and chopped
4 garlic cloves, peeled and minced
8 ounces shrimp, peeled, deveined, and chopped
2 cups chicken stock
1 tablespoon coconut milk
½ cup fresh parsley, chopped
For the flounder:
4 flounder fillets
2 tablespoons butter

Directions:
1.In a bowl, mix all the ingredients for the seasoning and stir. Reserve 2 tablespoons of mixture, rub the flounder with the remainder and set aside. Heat a pan over medium heat, add bacon, stir, and cook for 6 minutes.
2.Add celery, bell pepper, shallots, and 1 tablespoon butter, stir, and cook for 4 minutes.
3.Add tomato and garlic, stir, and cook for 4 minutes. Add coconut flour and reserved seasoning, stir, and cook for 2 minutes. Add chicken stock and bring to a simmer.
4.Heat another pan with 2 tablespoons butter over medium–high heat, add fish, cook for 2 minutes, flip, and cook for 2 minutes.
5.Add shrimp to pan with stock, stir, and cook for 2 minutes.
6.Add parsley, salt, pepper, coconut milk, stir, and take off the heat.
7.Divide fish on plates, top with the shrimp sauce, and serve.

Nutrition: Calories: 623, Fat: 31.9, Fiber: 3.6, Carbohydrates: 13.2, Protein: 67.3

Baked Calamari and Shrimp

Prep Time: 10 minutes **Cook Time:** 20 minutes
Servings: 1

Ingredients:
8 ounces calamari, cut into medium rings
7 ounces shrimp, peeled and deveined
1 eggs
3 tablespoons coconut flour
1 tablespoon coconut oil
2 tablespoons avocado, chopped
1 teaspoon tomato paste
1 tablespoon mayonnaise
A splash of Worcestershire sauce
1 teaspoon lemon juice
2 lemon slices
Salt and ground black pepper, to taste
½ teaspoon turmeric

Directions:
1.In a bowl, whisk egg with coconut oil. Add calamari rings and shrimp and toss to coat.
2.In another bowl, mix flour with salt, pepper, and turmeric and stir.
3.Coat the calamari and shrimp in mixture, place everything on a lined baking sheet, place in an oven at 400ºF, and bake for 10 minutes.
4.Flip calamari and shrimp and bake for 10 minutes.
5.In a bowl, mix avocado with mayonnaise and tomato paste, and mash using a fork.
6.Add Worcestershire sauce, lemon juice, salt, pepper, and stir well.
7.Divide calamari and shrimp on plates and serve with the sauce and lemon slices on the side.

Nutrition: Calories: 2022, Fat: 86.1, Fiber: 9.2, Carbohydrates: 129.6, Protein: 163.8

Fiery Oysters

Prep Time: 10 minutes **Cook Time:** 0 minutes
Servings: 4

Ingredients:
12 oysters, shucked
Juice of 2 lemons
Juice from 1 lime
Zest from 2 limes
1 Serrano chili pepper, chopped
1 cup tomato juice
½ teaspoon fresh ginger, grated
¼ teaspoon garlic, minced
Salt, to taste
¼ cup olive oil
¼ cup fresh cilantro, chopped
¼ cup scallions, chopped

Directions:
1.In a bowl, mix lemon juice, lime juice, lime zest, chili pepper, tomato juice, ginger, garlic, oil, scallions, cilantro, salt, and stir well.
2.Spoon this onto oysters and serve them.

Nutrition: Calories: 179, Fat: 14.6, Fiber: 0.5, Carbohydrates: 6.4, Protein: 7.1

Shrimp Salad

Prep Time: 10 minutes **Cook Time:** 10 minutes
Servings: 4

Ingredients:
2 tablespoons olive oil
1 pound shrimp, peeled and deveined
Salt and ground black pepper, to taste
2 tablespoons lime juice

3 endives, leaves separated

3 tablespoons fresh parsley, chopped
2 teaspoons fresh mint, chopped
1 tablespoon fresh tarragon, chopped
1 tablespoon lemon juice
2 tablespoons mayonnaise
1 teaspoon lime zest
½ cup sour cream

Directions:
1.In a bowl, mix shrimp with salt, pepper, olive oil, toss to coat, and spread them on a lined baking sheet.
2.Place shrimp in the oven at 400ºF and bake for 10 minutes.
3.Add shrimp to a bowl with lime juice, toss them to coat, and set aside.
4.In a bowl, mix mayonnaise with sour cream, lime zest, lemon juice, salt, pepper, tarragon, mint, parsley, and stir well.
5.Chop shrimp, add to salad dressing, toss to coat everything, spoon into the endive leaves, and serve.

Nutrition: Calories: 332, Fat: 18, Fiber: 8.1, Carbohydrates: 14.2, Protein: 30.2

Salmon Rolls

Prep Time: 10 minutes **Cook Time:** 0 minutes
Servings: 12

Ingredients:
2 nori sheets
1 small avocado, pitted, peeled, and diced
6 ounces smoked salmon, sliced
4 ounces cream cheese
1 cucumber, sliced
1 teaspoon wasabi paste
Pickled ginger, for serving

Directions:
1.Place nori sheets on a sushi mat.
2.Divide salmon slices avocado, and cucumber slices on them. In a bowl, mix cream cheese with wasabi paste and stir well.
3.Spread over cucumber slices, roll the nori sheets, press well, cut each into 6 pieces, and serve with pickled ginger.

Nutrition: Calories: 89, Fat: 7.2, Fiber: 1.4, Carbohydrates: 2.6, Protein: 4

Grilled Shrimp

Prep Time: 20 minutes **Cook Time:** 10 minutes
Servings: 4

Ingredients:
1 pound shrimp, peeled and deveined
1 tablespoon lemon juice
1 garlic clove, peeled and minced
½ cup fresh basil leaves
1 tablespoon pine nuts, toasted
2 tablespoons Parmesan cheese, grated
2 tablespoons olive oil
Salt and ground black pepper, to taste

Directions:
1.In a food processor, mix Parmesan cheese with basil, garlic, pine nuts, oil, salt, pepper, lemon juice, and blend well.
2.Transfer to a bowl, add shrimp, toss to coat, and set aside for 20 minutes.
3.Thread skewers with marinated shrimp, place on preheated grill over medium–high heat, cook for 3 minutes, flip, and cook for 3 minutes.
4.Arrange on plates and serve.

Nutrition: Calories: 234, Fat: 11.9, Fiber: 0.2, Carbohydrates: 2.7, Protein: 28.5

Calamari Salad

Prep Time: 30 minutes **Cook Time:** 4 minutes
Servings: 8

Ingredients:
2 long red chilies, chopped
2 small red chilies, chopped
2 garlic cloves, peeled and minced
3 green onions, chopped
1 tablespoon balsamic vinegar
Salt and ground black pepper, to taste
Juice of 1 lemon
6 pounds calamari hoods, tentacles set aside
3. 5 ounces olive oil
3 ounces arugula, for serving

Directions:
1.In a bowl, mix red chilies, green onions, vinegar, garlic, salt, pepper, lemon juice, half of the oil, and stir well.
2.Place calamari and tentacles in a bowl, season with salt, and pepper, drizzle remaining oil, toss to coat, and place on preheated grill pan over medium–high heat.
3.Cook for 2 minutes on each side, and transfer to the chili marinade.
4.Toss to coat, and set aside for 30 minutes.
5.Arrange arugula on plates, top with the calamari and its marinade, and serve.

Nutrition: Calories: 1288, Fat: 72.5, Fiber: 4.8, Carbohydrates: 78.5, Protein: 73

Cod Salad

Prep Time: 2 hours and 10 minutes **Cook Time:** 20 minutes
Servings: 8

Ingredients:
2 cups jarred pimiento peppers, chopped
2 pounds salt cod
1 cup fresh parsley, chopped
1 cup Kalamata olives, pitted and chopped
6 tablespoons capers
¾ cup olive oil
Salt and ground black pepper, to taste
Juice from 2 lemons
4 garlic cloves, peeled and minced
2 celery stalks, chopped
½ teaspoon red chili flakes
1 escarole head, leaves separated

Directions:
1.Put cod in a saucepan, add water to cover, bring to a boil over medium heat, boil for 20 minutes, drain, and cut into medium chunks.
2.Put cod in a salad bowl, add peppers, parsley, olives, capers, celery, garlic, lemon juice, salt, pepper, olive oil, chili flakes, and toss to coat.
3.Arrange the escarole leaves on a platter, add cod salad, and serve.

Nutrition: Calories: 342, Fat: 22.1, Fiber: 2.2, Carbohydrates: 3.6, Protein: 33.1

Swordfish with Peach Salsa

Prep Time: 10 minutes **Cook Time:** 6 minutes
Servings: 2

Ingredients:
2 medium swordfish steaks
Salt and ground black pepper, to taste
2 teaspoons avocado oil
1 tablespoon fresh cilantro, chopped
2 peaches, stoned, chopped
1 avocado, pitted, peeled, and chopped
A pinch of cumin
A pinch of onion powder
A pinch of garlic powder
1 orange, peeled and sliced
½ balsamic vinegar

Directions:
1.Season the fish steaks with salt, pepper, garlic powder, onion powder, and cumin.
2.Heat a pan with half of the oil over medium–high heat, add fish steaks, and cook them for 3 minutes on each side.
3.In a bowl, mix avocado with peaches, cilantro, balsamic vinegar, salt, pepper, and remaining oil and stir well.
4.Divide fish on plates, top with peach salsa and serve with orange slices on the side.

Nutrition: Calories: 794, Fat: 52.4, Fiber: 19.9, Carbohydrates: 45.2, Protein: 40.6

Grilled Swordfish

Prep Time: 3 hours and 10 minutes **Cook Time:** 10 minutes
Servings: 4

Ingredients:
1 tablespoon fresh parsley, chopped
1 lemon, cut into wedges
4 swordfish steaks
3 garlic cloves, peeled and minced
⅓ cup chicken stock
3 tablespoons olive oil
¼ cup lemon juice
Salt and ground black pepper, to taste
½ teaspoon dried rosemary
½ teaspoon dried sage
½ teaspoon dried marjoram

Directions:
1.In a bowl, mix chicken stock with garlic, lemon juice, olive oil, salt, pepper, sage, marjoram, rosemary, and whisk.
2.Add swordfish steaks, toss to coat, and keep in the refrigerator for 3 hours.
3.Place marinated fish steaks on preheated grill pan over medium–high heat, and cook for 5 minutes on each side.
4.Arrange on plates, sprinkle parsley onto fish, and serve with lemon wedges on the side.

Nutrition: Calories: 349, Fat: 18.9, Fiber: 0.6, Carbohydrates: 2.5, Protein: 40.9

Sushi Bowl

Prep Time: 10 minutes **Cook Time:** 7 minutes
Servings: 4

Ingredients:
1 ahi tuna steak
2 tablespoons coconut oil
1 cauliflower head, separated into florets
2 tablespoons green onions, chopped
1 avocado, pitted, peeled, and chopped
1 cucumber, grated
1 nori sheet, torn
Bean sprouts
For the salad dressing:
1 tablespoon sesame oil
2 tablespoons coconut aminos
1 tablespoon apple cider vinegar
A pinch of salt
1 teaspoon stevia

Directions:
1.Put cauliflower florets in a food processor and blend until you obtain a cauliflower "rice".
2.Put some water in a pot, put a steamer basket inside, add cauliflower rice, bring to a boil over medium heat, cover, steam for a few minutes, drain, and transfer "rice" to a bowl.
3.Heat a pan with coconut oil over medium–high heat, add tuna, cook for 1 minute on each side, and transfer to a cutting board.
4.Divide cauliflower rice into bowls, top nori pieces, sprouts, cucumber, green onions, and avocado.
5.In a bowl, mix sesame oil with vinegar, coconut aminos, salt, stevia, and whisk.
6.Drizzle over cauliflower rice and mixed vegetables, top with tuna pieces, and serve.

Nutrition: Calories: 239, Fat: 17.1, Fiber: 5.5, Carbohydrates: 11.5, Protein: 12.8

Poultry

Mexican Chicken Soup

Prep Time: 10 minutes **Cook Time:** 4 hours
Servings: 6

Ingredients:
1½ pounds chicken tights, skinless, boneless, and cubed
15 ounces chicken stock
15 ounces tomato passata
8 ounces Monterey jack

Directions:
1.In a slow cooker, mix chicken with stock, tomato passata, cheese, stir, cover, and cook on high for 4 hours.
2.Uncover slow cooker, stir soup, divide into bowls, and serve.

Nutrition: Calories: 397, Fat: 27.7, Fiber: 0, Carbohydrates: 4.2, Protein: 34.4

Chicken Gumbo

Prep Time: 10 minutes **Cook Time:** 7 hours
Servings: 5

Ingredients:
2 sausages, sliced
3 chicken breasts, cubed
2 tablespoons dried oregano
2 bell peppers, seeded and chopped
1 onion, peeled and chopped
28 ounces canned diced tomatoes
3 tablespoons dried thyme
2 tablespoons garlic powder
2 tablespoons dry mustard
1 teaspoon cayenne powder
1 tablespoons chili powder
Salt and ground black pepper, to taste
6 tablespoons Creole seasoning

Directions:
1.In a slow cooker, mix sausages with chicken, salt, pepper, bell peppers, oregano, onion, thyme, garlic powder, dry mustard, tomatoes, cayenne, chili, and Creole seasoning.
2.Cover and cook on low for 7 hours.
3.Uncover slow cooker again, stir the gumbo, and divide into bowls. Serve hot.

Nutrition: Calories: 445, Fat: 20.7, Fiber: 3.8, Carbohydrates: 13, Protein: 50.9

Chicken Thighs with Mushrooms and Cheese

Prep Time: 10 minutes **Cook Time:** 45 minutes
Servings: 4

Ingredients:
3 tablespoons butter
8 ounces mushrooms, sliced
2 tablespoons gruyere cheese, grated
Salt and ground black pepper, to taste
2 garlic cloves, peeled and minced
6 chicken thighs

Directions:
1.Heat a pan with 1 tablespoon butter over medium heat, add chicken thighs, season with salt and pepper, cook for 3 minutes on each side, and arrange in a baking dish.
2.Heat the pan again with the rest of the butter over medium heat, add garlic, stir, and cook for 1 minute.
3.Add mushrooms and stir well. Add salt and pepper, stir, and cook for 10 minutes.
4.Spoon mixture over chicken, sprinkle with cheese, place in an oven at 350ºF, and bake for 30 minutes.
5.Turn on oven's broiler, and broil everything for a 2 minutes. Divide on plates and serve.

Nutrition: Calories: 729, Fat: 34.2, Fiber: 0.6, Carbohydrates: 2.4, Protein: 98

Pepperoni Chicken Bake

Prep Time: 10 minutes **Cook Time:** 55 minutes
Servings: 6

Ingredients:
14 ounces tomato passata
1 tablespoon coconut oil
4 medium chicken breasts, skinless and boneless
Salt and ground black pepper, to taste
1 teaspoon dried oregano
6 ounces mozzarella cheese, sliced
1 teaspoon garlic powder
2 ounces pepperoni, sliced

Directions:
1.Put tomato paste in a small saucepan, bring to a boil over medium heat, simmer for 3 minutes, and take off the heat.
2.In a bowl, mix chicken with salt, pepper, garlic powder, oregano, and stir.
3.Heat a pan with coconut oil over medium–high heat, add chicken pieces, cook for 2 minutes on each side, and transfer to a baking dish.
4.Add mozzarella cheese slices on top, spread sauce, top with pepperoni slices, place in an oven at 400ºF, and bake for 30 minutes. Divide on plates and serve.

Nutrition: Calories: 491, Fat: 24.4, Fiber: 0.2, Carbohydrates: 4.7, Protein: 60.3

Fried Chicken

Prep Time: 24 hours **Cook Time:** 20 minutes
Servings: 4

Ingredients:
3 chicken breasts, cut into strips
4 ounces pork rinds, crushed
2 cups coconut oil
16 ounces jarred pickle juice
2 eggs, whisked

Directions:
1.In a bowl, mix chicken breast pieces with pickle juice, stir, cover, and keep in refrigerator for 24 hours.
2.Put eggs in a bowl, and pork rinds in another one.
3.Dip chicken pieces in egg, and then in pork rinds, and coat well.
4.Heat a pan with oil over medium–high heat, add chicken pieces, fry them for 3 minutes on each side, transfer to paper towels, drain grease, and serve.

Nutrition: Calories: 1488, Fat: 134.8, Fiber: 0, Carbohydrates: 2.4, Protein: 73.8

Simple Chicken Stir–fry

Prep Time: 10 minutes **Cook Time:** 12 minutes
Servings: 2

Ingredients:
2 chicken thighs, skinless, boneless, and cut into thin strips
1 tablespoon sesame oil
1 teaspoon red pepper flakes
1 teaspoon onion powder
1 tablespoon fresh ginger, grated
¼ cup tamari sauce
½ teaspoon garlic powder
½ cup water
1 tablespoon stevia
½ teaspoon xanthan gum
½ cup scallions, chopped
2 cups broccoli florets

Directions:
1.Heat a pan with oil over medium–high heat, add chicken and ginger, stir and cook for 3 minutes.
2.Add water, tamari sauce, onion powder, garlic powder, stevia, pepper flakes, xanthan gum, stir, and cook for 5 minutes.
3.Add broccoli and scallions, stir, cook for 2 minutes, and divide on plates. Serve hot.

Nutrition: Calories: 392, Fat: 19.1, Fiber: 3.6, Carbohydrates: 11.3, Protein: 43.9

Chicken Calzone

Prep Time: 10 minutes **Cook Time:** 1 hour
Servings: 12

Ingredients:
2 eggs
½ cup Parmesan cheese, grated
1 pound chicken breasts, skinless, boneless, and each sliced in half
½ cup keto marinara sauce
1 teaspoon Italian seasoning
1 teaspoon onion powder
1 teaspoon garlic powder
Salt and ground black pepper, to taste
¼ cup flaxseed, ground
8 ounces provolone cheese
For pizza crust:
4 eggs
6 oz. shredded mozzarella

Directions:
1.In a bowl, mix the Italian seasoning with onion powder, garlic powder, salt, pepper, flaxseed, and Parmesan cheese, and stir well.
2.In another bowl, mix eggs with a pinch of salt, and pepper, and whisk.
3.Dip chicken pieces in eggs, and then in seasoning mixture, place all pieces on a lined baking sheet, and bake in oven at 350ºF for 30 minutes.
4.For pizza crust crack eggs in a bowl, add cheese, mix well and spread the mixture on a baking sheet lined with parchment paper. Bake at 350°F for 3 minutes.
5.Put pizza crust on a lined baking sheet and spread half of provolone cheese on half. Take chicken out of oven, chop it, and spread over provolone cheese.
6.Add marinara sauce and then rest of the cheese.
7.Cover with other half of the dough and shape calzone.
8.Seal edges, place in an oven at 350ºF, and bake for 20 minutes. Let calzone cool down before slicing and serving.

Nutrition: Calories: 247, Fat: 14.9, Fiber: 0.7, Carbohydrates: 2.4, Protein: 25.2

Pecan-crusted Chicken

Prep Time: 10 minutes **Cook Time:** 20 minutes
Servings: 4

Ingredients:
1 egg, whisked
Salt and ground black pepper, to taste
3 tablespoons coconut oil
1½ cups pecans, chopped
4 chicken breasts

Directions:
1.Put pecans in a bowl and whisked egg in another.
2.Season chicken, dip in egg and then in pecans.
3.Heat a pan with oil over medium–high heat, add chicken, and cook until brown on both sides.
4.Transfer chicken pieces to a baking sheet, place in oven, and bake at 350ºF for 10 minutes. Divide on plates and serve.

Nutrition: Calories: 930, Fat: 65.2, Fiber: 5.3, Carbohydrates: 7.1, Protein: 80.6

Lemon Chicken

Prep Time: 10 minutes **Cook Time:** 45 minutes
Servings: 6

Ingredients:
1 whole chicken, cut into medium–sized pieces
Salt and ground black pepper, to taste
Juice from 2 lemons
Zest from 2 lemons
Lemon rinds from 2 lemons

Directions:
1.Put chicken pieces in a baking dish, season with salt and pepper, and drizzle lemon juice.
2.Toss to coat well, add lemon zest, and lemon rinds, place in an oven at 375ºF, and bake for 45 minutes.
3.Discard lemon rinds, divide chicken onto plates, drizzle sauce from baking dish and serve.

Nutrition: Calories: 328, Fat: 12.7, Fiber: 0.4, Carbohydrates: 1.3, Protein: 49.4

Chicken Meatloaf

Prep Time: 10 minutes **Cook Time:** 40 minutes
Servings: 8

Ingredients:
1 cup tomato sauce
1 teaspoon minced garlic
1 teaspoon dried basil
1⁄2 teaspoon dried rosemary
2 pound ground chicken
2 tablespoons fresh parsley, chopped
4 garlic cloves, peeled and minced
2 teaspoons onion powder
2 teaspoons Italian seasoning
Salt and ground black pepper, to taste
For the filling:
½ cup ricotta cheese
1 cup Parmesan cheese, grated
1 cup mozzarella cheese, shredded
2 teaspoons fresh chives, chopped
2 tablespoons fresh parsley, chopped
1 garlic clove, peeled and minced

Directions:
1.In a bowl, mix chicken with half of tomato paste, garlic, basil, rosemary, salt, pepper, Italian seasoning, 4 garlic cloves, onion powder, 2 tablespoons parsley, and stir well.
2.In another bowl, mix ricotta cheese with half of Parmesan cheese, half of mozzarella cheese, chives, 1 garlic clove, salt, pepper, 2 tablespoons parsley, and stir well.
3.Put half of chicken mix into a loaf pan and spread evenly.
4.Add cheese filling and spread evenly. Top with rest of meat and spread again.
5.Place meatloaf in oven at 400ºF and bake for 20 minutes.
6.Take meatloaf out of oven, spread rest of tomato paste, garlic, basil, rosemary, rest of the cheese, and bake for 20 minutes.
7.Allow meatloaf to cool, slice, divide on plates, and serve.

Nutrition: Calories: 334, Fat: 15.6, Fiber: 0.5, Carbohydrates: 3.7, Protein: 43.9

Chicken with Green Onion Sauce

Prep Time: 10 minutes **Cook Time:** 27 minutes
Servings: 4

Ingredients:
2 tablespoons butter
1 green onion, peeled and chopped
4 chicken breast halves, skinless and boneless
Salt and ground black pepper, to taste
8 ounces sour cream

Directions:
1.Heat a pan with butter over medium–high heat, add chicken pieces, season with salt and pepper, cover, reduce heat, and simmer for 10 minutes.
2.Uncover pan, turn chicken pieces, and cook covered for 10 minutes.
3.Add green onions, stir, and cook for 2 minutes.
4.Take off heat, add more salt, and pepper if needed, add sour cream, stir well, cover pan, and set aside for 5 minutes. Stir again, divide on plates, and serve.

Nutrition: Calories: 659, Fat: 36.6, Fiber: 0.1, Carbohydrates: 2.7, Protein: 75.8

Chicken Meatballs

Prep Time: 10 minutes **Cook Time:** 15 minutes
Servings: 3

Ingredients:
1 pound ground chicken
Salt and ground black pepper, to taste
2 tablespoons plain yogurt
½ cup almond flour
¼ cup cheddar cheese, grated
¼ cup tomato paste more for serving
3 teaspoons cayenne pepper powder
1 egg

Directions:
1.In a bowl, mix chicken meat with salt, pepper, yogurt, flour, cheddar cheese, tomato paste, cayenne pepper, egg, and stir well.
2.Shape 9 meatballs, place on a lined baking sheet, and bake at 500ºF for 15 minutes.
3.Serve chicken meatballs with hot sauce on the side.

Nutrition: Calories: 461, Fat: 19.2, Fiber: 5.4, Carbohydrates: 18.7, Protein: 52.2

One-pot Roasted Chicken

Prep Time: 10 minutes **Cook Time:** 40 minutes
Servings: 12

Ingredients:
1 whole chicken
½ teaspoon onion powder
½ teaspoon garlic powder
Salt and ground black pepper, to taste
2 tablespoons coconut oil
1 teaspoon Italian seasoning
1½ cups chicken stock
2 teaspoons guar gum

Directions:
1.Rub chicken with half of oil, garlic powder, salt, pepper, Italian seasoning, and onion powder. Put rest of oil into an Instant Pot, andadd chicken to pot.
2.Add stock, cover Instant Pot, and cook on Poultry mode for 40 minutes.
3.Transfer chicken to a platter and set aside.
4.Set instant pot on Sauté mode, add guar gum, stir, and cook until it thickens. Pour sauce over chicken and serve.

Nutrition: Calories: 463, Fat: 31.8, Fiber: 0, Carbohydrates: 0.4, Protein: 44.1

Spinach and Artichoke Chicken

Prep Time: 10 minutes **Cook Time:** 50 minutes
Servings: 4

Ingredients:
4 ounces cream cheese
4 chicken breasts
10 ounces canned artichoke hearts, chopped
10 ounces spinach
½ cup Parmesan cheese, grated
1 tablespoon onion powder
1 tablespoon garlic powder
Salt and ground black pepper, to taste
4 ounces mozzarella cheese, shredded

Directions:
1.Place chicken breasts on a lined baking sheet, season with salt, pepper, place in an oven at 400°F and bake for 30 minutes.
2.In a bowl, mix artichokes with onion, cream cheese, Parmesan cheese, spinach, garlic, salt, pepper, and stir.
3.Take chicken out of oven, cut each piece in the middle, divide artichokes mixture, sprinkle with mozzarella cheese, place in an oven at 400°F and bake for 15 minutes. Serve hot.

Nutrition: Calories: 573, Fat: 30.6, Fiber: 5.4, Carbohydrates: 12.5, Protein: 63.5

Chicken-stuffed Mushrooms

Prep Time: 10 minutes **Cook Time:** 10 minutes
Servings: 6

Ingredients:
10 ounces button mushroom caps
4 ounces cream cheese
¼ cup butternut squash, chopped
1 teaspoon plain yogurt
4 tablespoons hot sauce
¾ cup blue cheese, crumbled
¼ cup onion, chopped
½ cup chicken meat, already cooked and chopped
Salt and ground black pepper, to taste
Vegetable oil cooking spray

Directions:
1.In a bowl, mix cream cheese with blue cheese, hot sauce, yogurt, salt, pepper, chicken, squash, onion, and stir.
2.Stuff each mushroom cap with mixture, place on a lined baking sheet, spray with cooking spray, place in oven at 425°F and bake for 10 minutes.
3.Divide on plates and serve.

Nutrition: Calories: 167, Fat: 12.4, Fiber: 0.9, Carbohydrates: 4.3, Protein: 10.6

Chicken-stuffed Avocados

Prep Time: 10 minutes **Cook Time:** 0 minutes
Servings: 2

Ingredients:
2 avocados, cut in half and pitted
¼ cup mayonnaise
1 teaspoon dried thyme
2 tablespoons cream cheese
1½ cups chicken, cooked and shredded
Salt and ground black pepper, to taste
¼ teaspoon cayenne pepper
½ teaspoon onion powder
½ teaspoon garlic powder
1 teaspoon paprika
2 tablespoons lemon juice

Directions:
1.Scoop the inside of the avocado halves and put flesh in a bowl.
2.Put avocado cups to one side. Add chicken to avocado flesh and stir.
3.Add mayonnaise, thyme, cream cheese, cayenne, onion, garlic, paprika, salt, pepper, lemon juice, and stir well.
4.Stuff avocados with chicken mixture and serve.

Nutrition: Calories: 1142, Fat: 64.2, Fiber: 13.7, Carbohydrates: 24.9, Protein: 116.5

Chicken Nuggets

Prep Time: 10 minutes **Cook Time:** 15 minutes
Servings: 2

Ingredients:
½ cup coconut flour
1 egg
2 tablespoons garlic powder
2 chicken breasts, cubed
Salt and ground black pepper, to taste
½ cup butter

Directions:
1.In a bowl, mix garlic powder with coconut flour, salt, pepper, and stir. In another bowl, whisk egg well.
2.Dip chicken breast cubes in egg mixture, then in flour mixture.
3.Heat a pan with butter over medium heat, drop chicken nuggets and cook them for 5 minutes on each side.
4.Transfer to paper towels, drain grease, and then serve.

Nutrition: Calories: 1171, Fat: 74.9, Fiber: 13.3, Carbohydrates: 26.3, Protein: 94.1

Chicken Wings with Mint Chutney

Prep Time: 20 minutes **Cook Time:** 25 minutes
Servings: 6

Ingredients:
18 chicken wings, cut in half
1 tablespoon turmeric
1 tablespoon cumin
1 tablespoon fresh ginger, grated
1 tablespoon coriander
1 tablespoon paprika
A pinch of cayenne pepper
Salt and ground black pepper, to taste
2 tablespoons olive oil
For the chutney:
Juice of ½ lime
1 cup fresh mint leaves
1 small ginger piece, peeled and chopped
¾ cup cilantro
1 tablespoon olive oil
1 tablespoon water
Salt and ground black pepper, to taste
1 Serrano pepper

Directions:
1.In a bowl, mix 1 tablespoon ginger with cumin, coriander, paprika, turmeric, salt, pepper, cayenne, 2 tablespoons oil, and stir well.
2.Add chicken wings pieces to mixture, toss to coat well, and keep in the refrigerator for 20 minutes.
3.Heat a grill pan over high heat, add marinated wings, cook for 25 minutes, turning them from time to time, and transfer to a bowl.
4.In a blender, mix mint with cilantro, ginger, juice from ½ lime, 1 tablespoon olive oil, salt, pepper, water, Serrano pepper, and blend well.
5.Serve chicken wings with sauce on the side.

Nutrition: Calories: 452, Fat: 15.3, Fiber: 1.1, Carbohydrates: 2, Protein: 72.7

Grilled Chicken Wings

Prep Time: 2 hours and 10 minutes **Cook Time:** 15 minutes
Servings: 5

Ingredients:
2 pounds wings
Juice from 1 lime
½ cup fresh cilantro, chopped
2 garlic cloves, peeled and minced
1 jalapeño pepper, chopped
3 tablespoons coconut oil
Salt and ground black pepper, to taste
Lime wedges, for serving
Mayonnaise, for serving

Directions:
1.In a bowl, mix lime juice with cilantro, garlic, jalapeño, coconut oil, salt, and pepper, and whisk.
2.Add chicken wings, toss to coat, and keep in the refrigerator for 2 hours.
3.Place chicken wings on a preheated grill pan over medium–high heat, and cook for 7 minutes on each side.
4.Serve the chicken wings with mayonnaise and lime wedges.

Nutrition: Calories: 723, Fat: 51.8, Fiber: 0.2, Carbohydrates: 0.6, Protein: 60.3

Easy Baked Chicken

Prep Time: 10 minutes **Cook Time:** 20 minutes
Servings: 4

Ingredients:
4 bacon strips
4 chicken breasts
3 green onions, chopped
1 ounce coconut aminos
2 tablespoons coconut oil
4 ounces cheddar cheese, grated

Directions:
1.Heat a pan with the oil over high heat, add the chicken breasts, cook for 7 minutes, flip, and cook for 7 more minutes.
2.Heat another pan over medium–high heat, add bacon, cook until crispy, transfer to paper towels, drain grease and crumble.
3.Transfer chicken breast to a baking dish, add coconut aminos, crumbled bacon, cheese, and green onions on top, place in oven, set on broiler, and cook at a high temperature for 5 minutes. Divide on plates and serve.

Nutrition: Calories: 763, Fat: 40.1, Fiber: 0.3, Carbohydrates: 2.4, Protein: 92.8

Italian Chicken

Prep Time: 10 minutes **Cook Time:** 20 minutes
Servings: 4

Ingredients:
¼ cup olive oil
1 onion, peeled and chopped
4 chicken breasts, skinless and boneless
4 garlic cloves, peeled and minced
Salt and ground black pepper, to taste
½ cup green olives, pitted and chopped
4 anchovy fillets, chopped
1 tablespoon capers, chopped
1 pound tomatoes, cored and chopped
½ teaspoon red chili flakes

Directions:
1.Season chicken with salt, pepper, and rub with half of the oil.
2.Place into a preheated pan over high temperature, cook for 2 minutes, flip, and cook for 2 minutes.
3.Place chicken breasts in the oven at 450ºF and bake for 8 minutes.
4.Take chicken out of oven and divide on plates.
5.Heat the same pan with remaining oil over medium heat, add onion, garlic, olives, anchovies, chili flakes, capers, stir, and cook for 1 minute.
6.Add salt, pepper, tomatoes, stir, and cook for 2 minutes. Drizzle over chicken breasts and serve.

Nutrition: Calories: 733, Fat: 37.1, Fiber: 2.9, Carbohydrates: 9.8, Protein: 87.5

Fried Chicken with Paprika Sauce

Prep Time: 10 minutes **Cook Time:** 20 minutes
Servings: 5

Ingredients:
1 tablespoon coconut oil
3½ pounds chicken breasts
1 cup chicken stock
1¼ cups onion, peeled and chopped
1 tablespoon lime juice
¼ cup coconut milk
2 teaspoons paprika
1 teaspoon red pepper flakes
2 tablespoons green onions, chopped
Salt and ground black pepper, to taste

Directions:
1.Heat a pan with oil over medium–high heat, add chicken, cook for 2 minutes on each side, transfer to a plate, and set aside.
2.Reduce heat to medium, add onions to the pan, and cook for 4 minutes.
3.Add stock, coconut milk, pepper flakes, paprika, lime juice, salt, pepper, and stir well.
4.Return chicken to pan, add more salt, pepper, cover the pan, and cook for 15 minutes.
5.Divide on plates and serve.

Nutrition: Calories: 1031, Fat: 42.9, Fiber: 2.1, Carbohydrates: 7.8, Protein: 145.7

Skillet Chicken and Mushrooms

Prep Time: 10 minutes **Cook Time:** 30 minutes
Servings: 4

Ingredients:
4 chicken thighs
2 cups mushrooms, sliced
¼ cup butter
Salt and ground black pepper, to taste
½ teaspoon onion powder
½ teaspoon garlic powder
½ cup water
1 teaspoon Dijon mustard
1 tablespoon fresh tarragon, chopped

1.Directions:
2.Heat a pan with half of the butter over medium–high heat, add chicken thighs, season with salt, pepper, garlic powder, and onion powder, cook for 3 minutes on each side and transfer to a bowl.
3.Heat the same pan with remaining butter over medium–high heat, add mushrooms, stir, and cook for 5 minutes.
4.Add mustard and water and stir well. Return chicken pieces to pan, stir, cover, and cook for 15 minutes.
5.Add the tarragon, stir, cook for 5 minutes, divide on plates, and serve.

Nutrition: Calories: 664, Fat: 33.3, Fiber: 0.4, Carbohydrates: 1.2, Protein: 85.7

Chicken with Olive Tapenade

Prep Time: 10 minutes **Cook Time:** 10 minutes
Servings: 2

Ingredients:
1 chicken breast, cut into 4 pieces
2 tablespoons coconut oil
3 garlic cloves, peeled, and crushed
½ cup olive tapenade
For the tapenade:
1 cup black olives, pitted
Salt and ground black pepper, to taste
2 tablespoons olive oil
¼ cup fresh parsley, chopped
1 tablespoons lemon juice

Directions:
1.In a food processor, mix olives with salt, pepper, 2 tablespoons olive oil, lemon juice, and parsley, blend well, and transfer to a bowl.
2.Heat a pan with coconut oil over medium heat, add garlic, stir, and cook for 2 minutes.
3.Add chicken pieces and cook for 4 minutes on each side.
4.Divide chicken on plates and top with the olives tapenade.

Nutrition: Calories: 727, Fat: 61.6, Fiber: 2.5, Carbohydrates: 7.5, Protein: 37.7

Pan–seared Duck Breast

Prep Time: 10 minutes **Cook Time:** 20 minutes
Servings: 1

Ingredients:
1 medium duck breast, skin scored
1 tablespoon swerve
1 tablespoon heavy cream
2 tablespoons butter
½ teaspoon orange zest
Salt and ground black pepper, to taste
1 cup baby spinach
¼ teaspoon fresh sage

Directions:
1.Heat a pan with butter over medium heat. Once it melts, add swerve and stir until butter browns.
2.Add orange zest and sage, stir, and cook for 2 minutes. Add heavy cream and stir again.
3.Heat another pan over medium–high heat, add duck breast, skin side down, cook for 4 minutes, flip, and cook for another 3 minutes.
4.Pour orange sauce over duck breast, stir, and cook for a few minutes.
5.Add spinach to pan with the sauce, stir, and cook for 1 minute.
6.Take duck off heat, slice duck breast, and arrange on a plate.
7.Drizzle orange sauce on top and serve with the spinach on the side.

Nutrition: Calories: 1088, Fat: 54.3, Fiber: 0.7, Carbohydrates: 6.6, Protein: 142.2

Duck Breast with Vegetables

Prep Time: 10 minutes **Cook Time:** 10 minutes
Servings: 2

Ingredients:
2 duck breasts, skin on and sliced thin
2 zucchini, sliced
1 tablespoon coconut oil
1 green onion bunch, chopped
1 daikon, chopped
2 green bell peppers, seeded and chopped
Salt and ground black pepper, to taste

Directions:
1.Heat a pan with oil over medium–high heat, add green onions, stir, and cook for 2 minutes.
2.Add zucchini, daikon, bell peppers, salt, pepper, stir, and cook for 10 minutes.
3.Heat another pan over medium–high heat, add duck slices, cook for 3 minutes on each side, and transfer to pan with vegetables.
4.Cook for 3 minutes, divide on plates, and serve.

Nutrition: Calories: 558, Fat: 20.3, Fiber: 5.2, Carbohydrates: 19.3, Protein: 75.2

Duck Breast Salad

Prep Time: 10 minutes **Cook Time:** 15 minutes
Servings: 4

Ingredients:
1 tablespoon swerve
1 shallot, peeled and chopped
¼ cup red vinegar
¼ cup olive oil
¼ cup water
¾ cup raspberries
1 tablespoon Dijon mustard
Salt and ground black pepper, to taste
For the salad:
10 ounces baby spinach
2 medium duck breasts, boneless
4 ounces goats cheese, crumbled
Salt and ground black pepper, to taste
½ pint raspberries
½ cup pecans halves

Directions:
1.In a blender, mix the swerve with shallot, vinegar, water, oil, ¾ cup raspberries, mustard, salt, pepper, and blend well.
2.Strain into a bowl, and leave aside.
3.Score duck breast, season with salt, pepper, and place skin side down into a pan heated over medium–high heat.
4.Cook for 8 minutes, flip, and cook for 5 minutes.
5.Divide spinach on plates, sprinkle the goats cheese, pecan halves, and ½ pint raspberries.
6.Slice duck breasts and add on top of raspberries.
7.Drizzle raspberries vinaigrette on top and serve.

Nutrition: Calories: 628, Fat: 52, Fiber: 7.2, Carbohydrates: 15.1, Protein: 32

Turkey Pie

Prep Time: 10 minutes **Cook Time:** 40 minutes
Servings: 6

Ingredients:
2 cups turkey stock
1 cup turkey meat, cooked and shredded
Salt and ground black pepper, to taste
1 teaspoon fresh thyme, chopped
½ cup kale, chopped
½ cup butternut squash, peeled and chopped
½ cup cheddar cheese, shredded
¼ teaspoon paprika
¼ teaspoon garlic powder
¼ teaspoon xanthan gum
Vegetable oil cooking spray
For the crust:
¼ cup butter
¼ teaspoon xanthan gum
2 cups almond flour
A pinch of salt
1 egg
¼ cup cheddar cheese

Directions:
1. Heat a saucepan with the stock over medium heat. Add squash and turkey meat, stir, and cook for 10 minutes.
2. Add garlic powder, kale, thyme, paprika, salt, pepper, ½ cup cheddar cheese, and stir well. In a bowl, mix ¼ teaspoon xanthan gum with ½ cup stock from the pan, stir well, and add everything to the saucepan.
3. Take off heat and set aside. In a bowl, mix flour with ¼ teaspoon xanthan gum and a pinch of salt and stir.
4. Add butter, egg,¼ cup cheddar cheese, and stir until a pie crust dough forms. Shape into a ball and place in refrigerator.
5. Spray a baking dish with cooking spray and spread pie filling on the bottom.
6. Transfer dough to a working surface, roll into a circle, and top filling.
7. Press well, and seal edges, place in an oven at 350ºF, and bake for 35 minutes.
8. Let the pie to cool, and serve.

Nutrition: Calories: 241, Fat: 18.9, Fiber: 1.3, Carbohydrates: 4.9, Protein: 14

Chicken Fajitas

Prep Time: 10 minutes **Cook Time:** 15 minutes
Servings: 4

Ingredients:
2 pounds chicken breasts, skinless, boneless, and cut into strips
1 teaspoon garlic powder
1 teaspoon chili powder
2 teaspoons cumin
2 tablespoons lime juice
Salt and ground black pepper, to taste
1 teaspoon sweet paprika
2 tablespoons coconut oil
1 teaspoon coriander
1 green bell pepper, seeded and sliced
1 red bell pepper, seeded and sliced
1 onion, peeled and sliced
1 tablespoon fresh cilantro, chopped
1 avocado, pitted, peeled, and sliced
2 limes, cut into wedges

Directions:
1. In a bowl, mix lime juice with chili powder, cumin, salt, pepper, garlic powder, paprika, coriander, and stir.
2. Add chicken pieces and toss to coat well.
3. Heat a pan with half of the oil over medium–high heat, add chicken, cook for 3 minutes on each side, and transfer to a bowl.
4. Heat the pan with remaining oil over medium heat, add onion and bell peppers, stir, and cook for 6 minutes.
5. Return chicken to pan, add more salt, pepper, stir, and divide on plates.
6. Top with avocado, lime wedges, cilantro, and serve.

Nutrition: Calories: 643, Fat: 34, Fiber: 6.2, Carbohydrates: 17.2, Protein: 68.1

Turkey Soup

Prep Time: 10 minutes **Cook Time:** 30 minutes
Servings: 4

Ingredients:
3 celery stalks, chopped
1 onion, peeled and chopped
1 tablespoon butter
6 cups turkey stock
Salt and ground black pepper, to taste
¼ cup fresh parsley, chopped
3 cups baked spaghetti squash, chopped
3 cups turkey, cooked, and shredded

Directions:
1.Heat a pot with butter over medium–high heat, add celery and onion, stir, and cook for 5 minutes.
2.Add parsley, stock, turkey meat, salt, and pepper, stir, and cook for 20 minutes.
3.Add spaghetti squash, stir, and cook turkey soup for 10 minutes. Divide into bowls and serve.

Nutrition: Calories: 272, Fat: 8.5, Fiber: 2.5, Carbohydrates: 13.7, Protein: 33.6

Baked Turkey Delight

Prep Time: 10 minutes **Cook Time:** 45 minutes
Servings: 8

Ingredients:
4 cups zucchini, cut with a spiralizer
1 egg, whisked
3 cups cabbage, shredded
3 cups turkey meat, cooked and shredded
½ cup turkey stock
½ cup cream cheese
1 teaspoon poultry seasoning
2 cup cheddar cheese, grated
½ cup Parmesan cheese, grated
Salt and ground black pepper, to taste
¼ teaspoon garlic powder

Directions:
1.Heat a pan with stock over medium–low heat.
2.Add egg, cream, Parmesan cheese, cheddar cheese, salt, pepper, poultry seasoning, and garlic powder, stir, and bring to a gentle simmer.
3.Add turkey meat, cabbage, stir, and take off the heat.
4.Place zucchini noodles in a baking dish, add some salt and pepper, add the turkey mixture, and spread.
5.Cover with aluminum foil, place in an oven at 400ºF and bake for 35 minutes. Set aside to cool before serving.

Nutrition: Calories: 290, Fat: 18.5, Fiber: 1.3, Carbohydrates: 4.6, Protein: 26.4

Turkey Chili

Prep Time: 10 minutes **Cook Time:** 20 minutes
Servings: 8

Ingredients:
4 cups turkey meat, cooked and shredded
2 cups squash, chopped
6 cups chicken stock
Salt and ground black pepper, to taste
1 tablespoon canned chipotle peppers, chopped
½ teaspoon garlic powder
½ cup salsa verde
1 teaspoon coriander
2 teaspoons cumin
¼ cup sour cream
1 tablespoon fresh cilantro, chopped

Directions:
1.Heat a pan with stock over medium heat. Add squash, stir, and cook for 10 minutes.
2.Add turkey, chipotles, garlic powder, salsa verde, cumin, coriander, salt, pepper, stir, and cook for 10 minutes.
3.Add sour cream, stir, take off heat, and divide into bowls.
4.Top with some chopped cilantro and serve.

Nutrition: Calories: 153, Fat: 5.6, Fiber: 0.5, Carbohydrates: 2.9, Protein: 21.9

Turkey and Tomato Curry

Prep Time: 10 minutes **Cook Time:** 20 minutes
Servings: 4

Ingredients:
18 ounces turkey meat, minced
3 ounces spinach
20 ounces canned diced tomatoes
2 tablespoons coconut oil
2 tablespoons coconut cream
2 garlic cloves, peeled and minced
2 onions, peeled, and sliced
1 tablespoon coriander
2 tablespoons fresh ginger, grated
1 tablespoons turmeric
1 tablespoon cumin
Salt and ground black pepper, to taste
2 tablespoons chili powder

Directions:
1.Heat a pan with coconut oil over medium heat, add onion, stir, and cook for 5 minutes.
2.Add ginger and garlic, stir, and cook for 1 minute.
3.Add tomatoes, salt, pepper, coriander, cumin, turmeric, chili powder, and stir.
4.Add coconut cream, stir, and cook for 10 minutes.
5.Blend using an immersion blender and mix with spinach and turkey meat.
6.Bring to a simmer, cook for 15 minutes, and serve.

Nutrition: Calories: 240, Fat: 4, Fiber: 3, Carbohydrates: 2, Protein: 12

Turkey and Cranberry Salad

Prep Time: 10 minutes **Cook Time:** 0 minutes
Servings: 4

Ingredients:
4 cups romaine lettuce leaves, torn
2 cups turkey breast, cooked and cubed
1 lemon, peeled, and cut into small segments
3 tablespoons walnuts, chopped
3 kiwis, peeled and sliced
¼ cup cranberries
½ cup cranberry puree
1 cup lemon juice

Directions:
1.In a salad bowl, mix lettuce with turkey, lemon segments, apple pieces, cranberries, walnuts, and toss to coat.
2.In another bowl, mix cranberry puree and lemon juice, and stir.
3.Drizzle this over turkey salad, toss to coat, and serve with the kiwis on top.

Nutrition: Calories: 347, Fat: 15.4, Fiber: 3.6, Carbohydrates: 12.3, Protein: 40.1

Stuffed Chicken Breast

Prep Time: 10 minutes **Cook Time:** 15 minutes
Servings: 3

Ingredients:
8 ounces spinach, cooked, and chopped
3 chicken breasts
Salt and ground black pepper, to taste
4 ounces cream cheese, softened
3 ounces feta cheese, crumbled
1 garlic clove, peeled and minced
1 tablespoon coconut oil

Directions:
1.In a bowl, mix feta cheese with cream cheese, spinach, salt, pepper, garlic, and stir well.
2.Place chicken breasts on a working surface, cut a pocket in each, stuff them with spinach mixture, and season them with some salt and pepper.
3.Heat a pan the oil over medium–high heat, add stuffed chicken, cook for 5 minutes on each side, and place in the oven at 450ºF.
4.Bake for 10 minutes, divide on plates, and serve.

Nutrition: Calories: 912, Fat: 49.3, Fiber: 1.7, Carbohydrates: 5.2, Protein: 107.7

Chicken with Mustard Sauce

Prep Time: 10 minutes **Cook Time:** 30 minutes
Servings: 3

Ingredients:
8 bacon strips, chopped
⅓ cup Dijon mustard
Salt and ground black pepper, to taste
1 cup onion, chopped
1 tablespoon olive oil
1½ cups chicken stock
3 chicken breasts, skinless and boneless
¼ teaspoon sweet paprika

Directions:
1.In a bowl, mix paprika with mustard, salt, and pepper, and stir well. Spread this on chicken breasts and massage.
2.Heat a pan over medium–high heat, add bacon, stir, cook until it browns and transfer to a plate.
3.Heat the same pan with oil over medium–high heat, add chicken breasts, cook for 2 minutes on each side, transfer to a plate.
4.Heat pan once again over medium–high heat, add stock, stir, and bring to a simmer.
5.Add bacon and onions, salt, and pepper, and stir.
6.Return chicken to pan, stir gently, and simmer over medium heat for 20 minutes, turning meat halfway through.
7.Divide chicken on plates, drizzle the sauce over it, and serve.

Nutrition: Calories: 793, Fat: 36.9, Fiber: 1.8, Carbohydrates: 6.5, Protein: 103.6

Salsa Chicken

Prep Time: 10 minutes **Cook Time:** 1 hour and 15 minutes
Servings: 6

Ingredients:
6 chicken breasts, skinless and boneless
Salt and ground black pepper, to taste
1 cup cheddar cheese, shredded
Vegetable cooking spray
For keto salsa:
8 medium roasted tomatoes
2 chili peppers
4 cloves garlic
1 tablespoon salt
2 whole limes juiced

Directions:
1.Spray a baking dish with cooking oil, place chicken breasts on it, season with salt, pepper.
2.Combine all salsa ingredients in a blender, pulse well.
3.Cover chicken breasts with salsa. Place in an oven at 425ºF, and bake for 1 hour.
4.Spread cheese, and bake for 15 minutes.
5.Divide on plates and serve.

Nutrition: Calories: 788, Fat: 39.3, Fiber: 0.7, Carbohydrates: 18, Protein: 89.5

Creamy Chicken

Prep Time: 10 minutes **Cook Time:** 1 hour
Servings: 4

Ingredients:
4 chicken breasts, skinless and boneless
½ cup mayonnaise
½ cup sour cream
Salt and ground black pepper, to taste
¾ cup Parmesan cheese, grated
8 mozzarella cheese slices

Directions:
1.Spray a baking dish, place chicken breasts and top each piece with 2 mozzarella cheese slices.
2.In a bowl, mix Parmesan cheese with salt, pepper, mayonnaise, garlic powder, sour cream, and stir well.
3.Spread over the chicken, place the dish in the oven at 375ºF, and bake for 1 hour. Divide on plates and serve.

Nutrition: Calories: 925, Fat: 49.7, Fiber: 0, Carbohydrates: 10.6, Protein: 105

Italian Chicken

Prep Time: 10 minutes **Cook Time:** 1 hour
Servings: 6

Ingredients:
8 ounces mushrooms, chopped
1 pound Italian sausage, chopped
2 tablespoons avocado oil
6 cherry peppers, chopped
1 red bell pepper, seeded and chopped
1 onion, peeled and sliced
2 tablespoons garlic, minced
2 cups cherry tomatoes, halved
4 chicken thighs
Salt and ground black pepper, to taste
½ cup chicken stock
1 tablespoon balsamic vinegar
2 teaspoons dried oregano
Fresh parsley, chopped, for serving

Directions:
1.Heat a pan with half of the oil over medium heat, add sausages, stir, brown for a few minutes, and transfer to a plate.
2.Heat the pan again with remaining oil over medium heat, add chicken thighs, season with salt, and pepper, cook for 3 minutes on each side, and transfer to a plate.
3.Heat the pan again over medium heat, add cherry peppers, mushrooms, onion, and bell pepper, stir, and cook for 4 minutes.
4.Add garlic, stir, and cook for 2 minutes.
5.Add stock, vinegar, salt, pepper, oregano, cherry tomatoes, and stir.
6.Add chicken and sausages, stir gently, transfer everything to the oven at 400 degrees and bake for 30 minutes.
7.Sprinkle the parsley, divide on plates, and serve.

Nutrition: Calories: 673, Fat: 36.8, Fiber: 2, Carbohydrates: 8.7, Protein: 73.4

Chicken Casserole

Prep Time: 10 minutes **Cook Time:** 40 minutes
Servings: 8

Ingredients:
1½ pounds chicken breast, skinless, boneless, and cubed
1 egg
1 cup almond flour
¼ cup Parmesan cheese, grated
1½ teaspoons dried parsley
4 tablespoons avocado oil
4 cups spaghetti squash, already cooked
6 ounces mozzarella cheese, shredded
1½ cups tomato paste
1 teaspoon minced garlic
1 teaspoon dried basil
1⁄2 teaspoon dried rosemary
Fresh basil, chopped, for serving

Directions:
1.In a bowl, mix almond flour with Parmesan, salt, pepper, garlic powder, 1 teaspoon parsley, and stir. In another bowl, whisk egg with a pinch of salt and pepper.
2.Dip chicken in egg, and then in almond flour mixture.
3.Heat a pan with 3 tablespoons oil over medium–high heat, add chicken, cook until they are golden brown on both sides, and transfer to paper towels.
4.In a bowl, mix spaghetti squash with salt, pepper, dried basil, 1 tablespoon oil, and remaining parsley, and stir.
5.Spread this into a heatproof dish, add chicken pieces, and then tomato paste, minced garlic, dried basil and dried rosemary.
6.Top with shredded mozzarella cheese, place in an oven at 375ºF, and bake for 30 minutes.
7.Sprinkle with fresh basil at the end, set the casserole aside to cool, divide on plates, and serve.

Nutrition: Calories: 622, Fat: 16.3, Fiber: 8.1, Carbohydrates: 39.6, Protein: 82.3

Chicken–stuffed Peppers

Prep Time: 10 minutes **Cook Time:** 40 minutes
Servings: 3

Ingredients:
2 cups cauliflower florets
Salt and ground black pepper, to taste
1 onion, peeled and chopped
2 chicken breasts, skinless, boneless, cooked, and shredded
2 tablespoons fajita seasoning
1 tablespoon butter
6 bell peppers, tops cut off and seeds removed
⅔ cup water

Directions:
1.Put cauliflower florets in a food processor, add a pinch of salt and pepper, pulse well, and transfer to a bowl.
2.Heat a pan with butter over medium heat, add onions, stir, and cook for 2 minutes.
3.Add cauliflower, stir, and cook for 3 minutes.
4.Add seasoning, salt, pepper, water, and chicken, stir, and cook for 2 minutes.
5.Place bell peppers on a lined baking sheet, stuff each with chicken mixture, place in an oven at 350ºF, and bake for 30 minutes.
6.Divide them on plates and serve.

Nutrition: Calories: 532, Fat: 19, Fiber: 5.7, Carbohydrates: 29.2, Protein: 60.5

Chicken and Broccoli Casserole

Prep Time: 10 minutes **Cook Time:** 45 minutes
Servings: 4

Ingredients:
3 cups cheddar cheese, grated
10 ounces broccoli florets
3 chicken breasts, skinless, boneless, cooked, and cubed
1 cup mayonnaise
1 tablespoon coconut oil, melted
⅓ cup chicken stock
Salt and ground black pepper, to taste
Juice of 1 lemon

Directions:
1.Grease a baking dish with oil, and arrange chicken pieces on the bottom.
2.Spread broccoli florets, then half the cheese. In a bowl, mix mayo with stock, salt, pepper, and lemon juice.
3.Pour over the chicken, sprinkle rest of the cheese, cover dish with aluminum foil, and bake in the oven at 350ºF for 30 minutes.
4.Remove aluminum foil, and bake for 20 minutes. Serve hot.

Nutrition: Calories: 1041, Fat: 67.6, Fiber: 1.8, Carbohydrates: 19.9, Protein: 87

Creamy Chicken Soup

Prep Time: 10 minutes **Cook Time:** 20 minutes
Servings: 4

Ingredients:
3 tablespoons butter
4 ounces cream cheese
2 cups chicken meat, cooked and shredded
4 cups chicken stock
Salt and ground black pepper, to taste
½ cup sour cream
¼ cup celery, chopped

Directions:
1.In a blender, mix stock with red sauce, cream cheese, butter, salt, pepper, sour cream, and pulse well.
2.Transfer to a saucepan, heat over medium heat, add celery and chicken.
3.Stir, simmer for a few minutes, divide into bowls, and serve.

Nutrition: Calories: 381, Fat: 30.3, Fiber: 0.1, Carbohydrates: 2.9, Protein: 24.1

Chicken Crepes

Prep Time: 10 minutes **Cook Time:** 30 minutes
Servings: 8

Ingredients:
6 eggs
6 ounces cream cheese
1 teaspoon erythritol
1½ tablespoons coconut flour
⅓ cup Parmesan cheese, grated
A pinch of xanthan gum
Vegetable oil cooking spray
For the filling:
8 ounces spinach
8 ounces mushrooms, sliced
8 ounces rotisserie chicken, shredded
8 ounces cheese blend
2 ounces cream cheese
1 garlic clove, peeled and minced
1 onion, peeled and chopped
Liquids:
2 tablespoons red wine vinegar
2 tablespoons butter
½ cup heavy cream
1 teaspoon Worcestershire sauce
¼ cup chicken stock
A pinch of nutmeg
Fresh parsley, chopped

Directions:
1.In a bowl, mix 6 ounces cream cheese with eggs, Parmesan cheese, erythritol, xanthan, and coconut flour, and stir well until you obtain a crepe batter.
2.Heat a pan over medium heat, spray some cooking oil, pour some of the batter, spread well into the pan, cook for 2 minutes, flip, and cook for 30 seconds more. Repeat with rest of the batter and place all crepes on a plate.
3.Heat a pan with 2 tablespoon butter over medium–high heat, add onion, stir, and cook for 2 minutes.
4.Add garlic, stir, and cook for 1 minute. Add mushrooms, stir, and cook for 2 minutes. Add chicken, spinach, salt, pepper, stock, vinegar, nutmeg, Worcestershire sauce, heavy cream, cream cheese, and 6 ounces of cheese blend, stir, and cook for 7 minutes.
5.Fill each crepe with mixture, roll them, and arrange them all in a baking dish. Top with remaining cheese blend, place under a preheated broiler for a couple of minutes.
6.Divide crepes on plates, top with chopped parsley, and serve.

Nutrition: Calories: 372, Fat: 22.7, Fiber: 2.1, Carbohydrates: 23.9, Protein: 19.7

Crusted Chicken

Prep Time: 10 minutes **Cook Time:** 35 minutes
Servings: 4

Ingredients:
4 bacon slices, cooked and crumbled
4 chicken breasts, skinless and boneless
1 tablespoon water
½ cup avocado oil
1 egg, whisked
Salt and ground black pepper, to taste
1 cup Asiago cheese, shredded
¼ teaspoon garlic powder
1 cup Parmesan cheese, grated

Directions:
1.In a bowl, mix Parmesan cheese with garlic, salt, pepper, and stir.
2.Put whisked egg in another bowl and mix with the water.
3.Season chicken with salt, pepper, and dip each piece into egg, and then into cheese mixture.
4.Heat a pan with oil over medium–high heat, add chicken breasts, cook until golden on both sides, and transfer to a baking pan.
5.Place in an oven at 350ºF, and bake for 20 minutes.
6.Top chicken with bacon and Asiago cheese, place in an oven, turn on broiler, and broil for a couple of minutes. Serve hot.

Nutrition: Calories: 1065, Fat: 4, Fiber: 1.2, Carbohydrates: 3.1, Protein: 132.1

Four-cheese Chicken

Prep Time: 10 minutes **Cook Time:** 50 minutes
Servings: 4

Ingredients:
3 pounds chicken breasts
2 ounces muenster cheese, cubed
2 ounces cream cheese
4 ounces cheddar cheese, cubed
2 ounces provolone cheese, cubed
1 zucchini, shredded
Salt and ground black pepper, to taste
1 teaspoon garlic, minced
½ cup bacon, cooked and crumbled

Directions:
1.Season zucchini with salt and pepper, set aside for a few minutes, squeeze well, and transfer to a bowl.
2.Add bacon, garlic, more salt, pepper, cream cheese, cheddar cheese, Muenster cheese, and provolone cheese, and stir.
3.Cut slits into chicken breasts, season with salt, pepper, and stuff with zucchini and cheese mixture.
4.Place on a lined baking sheet, place in an oven at 400ºF, and bake for 45 minutes. Divide on plates and serve.

Nutrition: Calories: 1179, Fat: 67.6, Fiber: 0.6, Carbohydrates: 3.8, Protein: 131.8

Cheesy Chicken

Prep Time: 10 minutes **Cook Time:** 30 minutes
Servings: 4

Ingredients:
1 zucchini, chopped
Salt and ground black pepper, to taste
1 teaspoon garlic powder
1 tablespoon avocado oil
2 chicken breasts, skinless, boneless, and sliced
1 tomato, cored and chopped
½ teaspoon dried oregano
½ teaspoon dried basil
½ cup mozzarella cheese, shredded

Directions:
1.Season chicken with salt, pepper, and garlic powder.
2.Heat a pan with oil over medium heat, add chicken slices, brown on all sides, and transfer them to a baking dish.
3.Heat the pan again over medium heat, add zucchini, oregano, tomato, basil, salt, and pepper, stir, cook for 2 minutes and pour over chicken.
4.Place in an oven at 325ºF and bake for 20 minutes.
5.Spread mozzarella cheese over chicken, place in an oven again, and bake for 5 minutes. Divide on plates and serve.

Nutrition: Calories: 306, Fat: 12, Fiber: 1, Carbohydrates: 3.2, Protein: 44.2

Bacon-wrapped Chicken

Prep Time: 10 minutes **Cook Time:** 35 minutes
Servings: 4

Ingredients:
1 tablespoon fresh chives, chopped
8 ounces cream cheese
2 pounds chicken breasts, skinless and boneless
12 bacon slices
Salt and ground black pepper, to taste

Directions:
1.Heat a pan over medium heat, add bacon, cook until halfway done, transfer to paper towels and drain the grease.
2.In a bowl, mix cream cheese with salt, pepper, chives, and stir.
3.Use a meat tenderizer to flatten chicken breasts, add cream cheese mixture, roll them, and wrap each in a bacon slice.
4.Arrange wrapped chicken breasts into a baking dish, place in an oven at 375ºF and bake for 30 minutes.
5.Divide on plates and serve.

Nutrition: Calories: 937, Fat: 60.4, Fiber: 0, Carbohydrates: 2.4, Protein: 91

Orange Chicken

Prep Time: 10 minutes **Cook Time:** 15 minutes
Servings: 4

Ingredients:
2 pounds chicken thighs, skinless, boneless, and cut into pieces
Salt and ground black pepper, to taste
3 tablespoons coconut oil
¼ cup coconut flour
For the sauce:
2 tablespoons fish sauce
1½ teaspoons lemon zest
1 tablespoon fresh ginger, grated
¼ cup orange juice
2 teaspoons stevia
¼ teaspoon sesame seeds
2 tablespoons scallions, chopped
½ teaspoon coriander
1 cup water
¼ teaspoon red pepper flakes
2 tablespoons gluten–free soy sauce

Directions:
1.In a bowl, mix coconut flour, salt, pepper, and stir.
2.Add chicken pieces and toss to coat well.
3.Heat a pan with oil over medium heat, add chicken, cook until golden brown on both sides, and transfer to a bowl.
4.In a blender, mix lemon juice with ginger, fish sauce, soy sauce, stevia, lemon zest, water, coriander, and blend well.
5.Pour into a pan and heat over medium heat.
6.Add chicken, stir, and cook for 2 minutes.
7.Add sesame seeds, scallions, pepper flakes, stir cook for 2 minutes, and take off heat. Divide on plates and serve.

Nutrition: Calories: 542, Fat: 27.4, Fiber: 0.9, Carbohydrates: 4.3, Protein: 65

Chicken Pie

Prep Time: 10 minutes **Cook Time:** 45 minutes
Servings: 4

Ingredients:
½ cup onion, peeled and chopped
3 tablespoons butter
½ cup butternut squash, peeled and chopped
3 garlic cloves, peeled and minced
Salt and ground black pepper, to taste
¾ cup heavy cream
½ cup chicken stock
12 ounces chicken, cubed
2 tablespoons Dijon mustard
¾ cup cheddar cheese, shredded
For the dough:
¾ cup almond flour
3 tablespoons cream cheese
1½ cup mozzarella cheese, shredded
1 egg
1 teaspoon onion powder
1 teaspoon garlic powder
1 teaspoon Italian seasoning
Salt and ground black pepper, to taste

Directions:
1.Heat a pan with butter over medium heat, add onion, squash, garlic, salt, pepper, stir, and cook for 5 minutes.
2.Add chicken, stir, and cook for 3 minutes.
3.Add heavy cream, stock, salt, pepper, mustard, stir, and cook for 7 minutes.
4.Add cheddar cheese, stir well, take off heat, and keep warm.
5.In a bowl, mix mozzarella cheese with cream cheese, stir, and heat in a microwave for 1 minute.
6.Add garlic powder, Italian seasoning, salt, pepper, onion powder, flour, egg, and stir well. Knead dough well, divide into 4 pieces, and flatten each into a circle.
7.Divide chicken mix into 4 ramekins, top each with a dough circle, place in an oven at 375ºF for 25 minutes. Serve the chicken pies warm.

Nutrition: Calories: 645, Fat: 45.9, Fiber: 2.8, Carbohydrates: 9.2, Protein: 48

Chicken in Creamy Sauce

Prep Time: 10 minutes **Cook Time:** 1 hour and 10 minutes
Servings: 4

Ingredients:
8 chicken thighs
Salt and ground black pepper, to taste
1 onion, peeled and chopped
1 tablespoon coconut oil
4 bacon strips, chopped
4 garlic cloves, peeled and minced
10 ounces cremini mushrooms, halved
2 cups chardonnay
1 cup whipping cream
½ cup fresh parsley, chopped

Directions:
1.Heat a pan with oil over medium heat, add bacon, stir, cook until crispy, take off heat, and transfer to paper towels.
2.Heat the pan with bacon fat over medium heat, add chicken pieces, season with salt, and pepper, cook until brown, and transfer to paper towels.
3.Heat the pan again over medium heat, add onions, stir, and cook for 6 minutes.
4.Add garlic, stir, cook for 1 minute, and transfer next to bacon pieces.
5.Return pan to stove and heat again over medium temperature.
6.Add mushrooms, stir, and cook them for 5 minutes.
7.Return chicken, bacon, garlic and onion to pan.
8.Add wine, stir, bring to a boil, reduce heat, and simmer for 40 minutes.
9.Add parsley and cream, stir, and cook for 10 minutes. Divide on plates and serve.

Nutrition: Calories: 1044, Fat: 45.8, Fiber: 1.3, Carbohydrates: 9.6, Protein: 125.4

Savory Chicken

Prep Time: 10 minutes **Cook Time:** 1 hour
Servings: 4

Ingredients:
6 chicken breasts, skinless and boneless
Salt and ground black pepper, to taste
¼ cup jalapeños, chopped
5 bacon slices, chopped
8 ounces cream cheese
¼ cup onion, peeled and chopped
½ cup mayonnaise
½ cup Parmesan cheese, grated
1 cup cheddar cheese, grated
For the topping:
2 ounces pork skins, crushed
4 tablespoons melted butter
½ cup Parmesan cheese

Directions:
1.Arrange chicken breasts in a baking dish, season with salt, pepper, place in an oven at 425ºF and bake for 40 minutes.
2.Heat a pan over medium heat, add bacon, stir, cook until crispy and transfer to a plate.
3.Heat the pan again over medium heat, add onions, stir, and cook for 4 minutes.
4.Take off heat, add bacon, jalapeño, cream cheese, mayonnaise, cheddar cheese, and ½ cup Parmesan cheese, stir well, and spread over chicken.
5.In a bowl, mix pork skin with butter, and ½ cup Parmesan cheese, and stir.
6.Spread this over chicken as well, place in oven, and bake for 15 minutes. Serve hot.

Nutrition: Calories: 1452, Fat: 95.2, Fiber: 0.2, Carbohydrates: 11.2, Protein: 133.4

Chicken with Sour Cream Sauce

Prep Time: 10 minutes **Cook Time:** 40 minutes
Servings: 4

Ingredients:
4 chicken thighs
Salt and ground black pepper, to taste
1 teaspoon onion powder
¼ cup sour cream
2 tablespoons sweet paprika

Directions:
1.In a bowl, mix paprika with salt, pepper, onion powder, and stir.
2.Season chicken pieces with paprika mixture, arrange them on a lined baking sheet, and bake in the oven at 400ºF for 40 minutes.
3.Divide chicken on plates and set aside.
4.Pour juices from pan into a bowl and add sour cream. Stir sauce well and drizzle over chicken.

Nutrition: Calories: 526, Fat: 22.4, Fiber: 1.3, Carbohydrates: 2.5, Protein: 74.9

Red–hot Chicken Wings

Prep Time: 10 minutes **Cook Time:** 55 minutes
Servings: 4

Ingredients:
3 pounds chicken wings
Salt and ground black pepper, to taste
3 tablespoons coconut aminos
2 teaspoons white vinegar
3 tablespoons rice vinegar
3 tablespoons stevia
¼ cup scallions, chopped
½ teaspoon xanthan gum
5 dried chilies, chopped

Directions:
1.Spread chicken wings on a lined baking sheet, season with salt and pepper, place in an oven at 375ºF and bake for 45 minutes.
2.Heat a small pan over medium heat, add white vinegar, rice vinegar, coconut aminos, stevia, xanthan gum, scallions, chilies, stir well, bring to a boil, cook for 2 minutes, and take off heat.
3.Dip chicken wings into sauce, arrange them all on the baking sheet again, and bake for 10 minutes. Serve hot.

Nutrition: Calories: 815, Fat: 27.9, Fiber: 15.9, Carbohydrates: 36.8, Protein: 103.6

Chicken Stroganoff

Prep Time: 10 minutes **Cook Time:** 4 hours and 10 minutes
Servings: 4

Ingredients:
2 garlic cloves, peeled and minced
8 ounces mushrooms, chopped
¼ teaspoon celery seeds, ground
1 cup chicken stock
1 cup coconut milk
1 onion, peeled and chopped
1 pound chicken breasts, cut into medium–sized pieces
1½ teaspoons dried thyme
2 tablespoons fresh parsley, chopped
Salt and ground black pepper, to taste
4 zucchini, cut with a spiralizer

Directions:
1.Put the chicken in a slow cooker. Add salt, pepper, onion, garlic, mushrooms, coconut milk, celery seeds, stock, half of the parsley, and thyme.
2.Stir, cover, and cook on high for 4 hours. Uncover, add more salt and pepper if needed, and the rest of the parsley, and stir.
3.Heat a pan with water over medium heat, add some salt, bring to a boil, add the zucchini pasta, cook for 1 minute, and drain.
4.Divide on plates, add the chicken mixture on top, and serve.

Nutrition: Calories: 413, Fat: 23.4, Fiber: 4.7, Carbohydrates: 15.1, Protein: 38.9

Balsamic Chicken

Prep Time: 10 minutes **Cook Time:** 20 minutes
Servings: 4

Ingredients:
3 tablespoons coconut oil
2 pounds chicken breasts, skinless and boneless
3 garlic cloves, peeled and minced
Salt and ground black pepper, to taste
1 cup chicken stock
3 tablespoons stevia
½ cup balsamic vinegar
1 tomato, sliced thin
6 mozzarella slices
Fresh basil, chopped, for serving

Directions:
1.Heat a pan with oil over medium–high heat, add chicken pieces, season with salt and pepper, cook until brown on both sides and reduce heat.
2.Add garlic, vinegar, stock, stevia, stir, increase heat again, and cook for 10 minutes.
3.Transfer chicken breasts to a lined baking sheet, arrange mozzarella cheese slices on top, and top with basil.
4.Broil in the oven over medium heat until cheese melts and arrange tomato slices over chicken pieces. Divide on plates and serve.

Nutrition: Calories: 654, Fat: 34.7, Fiber: 0.2, Carbohydrates: 4.8, Protein: 78.1

Peanut–grilled Chicken

Prep Time: 10 minutes **Cook Time:** 20 minutes
Servings: 8

Ingredients:
2½ pounds chicken thighs, and drumsticks
1 tablespoon coconut aminos
1 tablespoon apple cider vinegar
A pinch of red pepper flakes
Salt and ground black pepper, to taste
½ teaspoon ground ginger
⅓ cup peanut butter
1 garlic clove, peeled and minced
½ cup warm water

Directions:
1.In a blender, mix peanut butter with water, aminos, salt, pepper, pepper flakes, ginger, garlic, vinegar, and blend well.
2.Pat chicken pieces dry, arrange in a pan, and pour peanut butter marinade over them.
3.Toss to coat and keep in refrigerator for 1 hour.
4.Place chicken pieces skin side down on a preheated grill pan over medium–high heat, cook for 10 minutes, flip, brush with some of marinade, and cook them for 10 minutes.
5.Divide on plates and serve.

Nutrition: Calories: 1196, Fat: 49.5, Fiber: 0.7, Carbohydrates: 2.4, Protein: 174.9

Chicken Stew

Prep Time: 10 minutes **Cook Time:** 2 hours
Servings: 4

Ingredients:
5 oz butternut squash, peeled and chopped
2 celery stalks, chopped
2 cups chicken stock
1 small onion, peeled and chopped
28 ounces chicken thighs, skinless, boneless, and cut into medium–sized pieces
3 garlic cloves, peeled and minced
½ teaspoon dried rosemary
1 cup spinach
½ teaspoon dried oregano
¼ teaspoon dried thyme
½ cup heavy cream
Salt and ground black pepper, to taste
A pinch of xanthan gum

Directions:
1.In a slow cooker, mix chicken with stock, celery, squash, onion, garlic, rosemary, thyme, oregano, some salt, pepper, stir, cover, and cook on high for 2 hours.
2.Add more salt and pepper, spinach, heavy cream, and stir.
3.Add xanthan gum, stir, and cook for 10 minutes. Divide into bowls and serve.

Nutrition: Calories: 464, Fat: 20.7, Fiber: 1.6, Carbohydrates: 8.1, Protein: 59.1

Chicken and Vegetable Stew

Prep Time: 10 minutes **Cook Time:** 30 minutes
Servings: 6

Ingredients:
2 cups whipping cream
40 ounces rotisserie chicken pieces, boneless, skinless, and shredded
3 tablespoons butter
½ cup onion, chopped
¾ cup red bell pepper, chopped
29 ounces canned chicken stock
Salt and ground black pepper, to taste
1 bay leaf
8 ounces mushrooms, chopped
1 cup chopped lettuce
17 ounces asparagus, trimmed
3 teaspoons fresh thyme, chopped

Directions:
1.Heat a pan with cream over medium heat, bring to a simmer, and cook until it's reduced.
2.Heat a pan with butter over medium heat, add onion and peppers, stir, and cook for 3 minutes.
3.Add stock, bay leaf, and some salt and pepper, bring to a boil, and simmer for 10 minutes.
4.Add asparagus, lettuce, mushrooms, stir, and cook for 7 minutes.
5.Add chicken pieces, stir, and cook for 3 minutes.
6.Add cream, thyme, salt and pepper to taste, stir, discard bay leaf, divide stew into bowls, and serve.

Nutrition: Calories: 920, Fat: 53.1, Fiber: 2.8, Carbohydrates: 18.4, Protein: 100.2

Chicken Pasta

Prep Time: 10 minutes **Cook Time:** 30 minutes
Servings: 4

Ingredients:
2 tablespoons butter
1 teaspoon garlic, minced
1 pound chicken cutlets
1 teaspoon Cajun seasoning
¼ cup scallions, chopped
½ cup tomatoes, cored and chopped
½ cup chicken stock
¼ cup whipping cream
½ cup cheddar cheese, grated
1 ounce cream cheese
¼ cup fresh cilantro, chopped
Salt and ground black pepper, to taste
For the pasta:
4 ounces cream cheese
8 eggs
Salt and ground black pepper, to taste
A pinch of garlic powder

Directions:
1.Heat a pan with 1 tablespoon butter over medium heat, add chicken cutlets, season with some Cajun seasoning, cook for 2 minutes on each side, and transfer to a plate.
2.Heat the pan with remaining butter over medium heat, add garlic, stir, and cook for 2 minutes.
3.Add tomatoes, stir, and cook for 2 minutes. Add stock and remaining Cajun seasoning, stir, and cook for 5 minutes.
4.Add whipping cream, cheddar cheese, 1 ounce cream cheese, salt, pepper, scallions, cilantro, stir well, cook for 2 minutes, and take off heat.
5.In a blender, mix 4 ounces cream cheese with eggs, salt, pepper, garlic powder, and pulse well.
6.Pour into a lined baking sheet, set aside for 5 minutes, and then bake in oven at 325ºF for 10 minutes.
7.Let pasta sheet cool down, transfer to a cutting board, roll, and cut into medium slices.
8.Divide pasta on plates, top with chicken mixture, and serve.

Nutrition: Calories: 602, Fat: 42.4, Fiber: 0.5, Carbohydrates: 3.5, Protein: 50.7

Red Meat Recipes

Thai Beef

Prep Time: 10 minutes **Cook Time:** 10 minutes
Servings: 6

Ingredients:
1 cup beef stock
4 tablespoons peanut butter
¼ teaspoon garlic powder
¼ teaspoon onion powder
1 tablespoon coconut aminos
1½ teaspoons lemon pepper
1 pound beef steak, cut into strips
Salt and ground black pepper, to taste
1 green bell pepper, seeded and chopped
3 green onions, chopped

Directions:
1.In a bowl, mix peanut butter with stock, aminos, lemon pepper, stir well and set aside.
2.Heat a pan over medium–high heat, add beef, season with salt, pepper, onion, garlic powder, and cook for 7 minutes.
3.Add green pepper, stir, and cook for 3 minutes.
4.Add peanut sauce and green onions, stir, cook for 1 minute, divide on plates, and serve.

Nutrition: Calories: 222, Fat: 10.3, Fiber: 1.6, Carbohydrates: 5.9, Protein: 26.6

Beef Patties

Prep Time: 10 minutes **Cook Time:** 35 minutes
Servings: 6

Ingredients:
½ cup cauliflower rice
1 egg
Salt and ground black pepper, to taste
1½ pounds ground beef
10 ounces canned onion soup
1 tablespoon coconut flour
¼ cup ketchup
3 teaspoons Worcestershire sauce
½ teaspoon dry mustard
¼ cup water

Directions:
1.In a bowl, mix ⅓ cup of onion soup with beef, salt, pepper, egg, cauliflower rice, and stir well.
2.Heat a pan over medium–high heat, shape 6 patties from beef mixture, place into the pan, and brown on both sides. In a bowl, mix rest of soup with coconut flour, water, dry mustard, Worcestershire sauce, ketchup, and stir well.
3.Pour over the beef patties, cover pan, and cook for 20 minutes stirring from occasionally. Divide on plates and serve.

Nutrition: Calories: 846, Fat: 28.2, Fiber: 1.4, Carbohydrates: 10.1, Protein: 130.3

Beef Pot Roast

Prep Time: 10 minutes **Cook Time:** 1 hour and 15 minutes
Servings: 4

Ingredients:
3½ pounds beef roast
4 ounces mushrooms, sliced
12 ounces beef stock
1 ounce onion powder
½ cup olive oil

Directions:
1.In a bowl, mix stock with onion powder, olive oil and stir.
2.Put beef roast in a pan, add mushrooms, stock mixture, cover with aluminum foil, place in an oven at 300ºF and bake for 1 hour and 15 minutes.
3.Allow roast to cool, slice, and serve with the gravy on top.

Nutrition: Calories: 990, Fat: 50.3, Fiber: 0.7, Carbohydrates: 6.7, Protein: 123

Jamaican Pork

Prep Time: 10 minutes **Cook Time:** 45 minutes
Servings: 12

Ingredients:
4 pounds pork shoulder
1 tablespoon coconut oil
½ cup beef stock
¼ cup Jamaican jerk spice mix

Directions:
1.Rub pork shoulder with Jamaican mixture, and place in an Instant Pot.
2.Add oil to pot, and set it to Sauté mode.
3.Add pork shoulder, and brown on all sides.
4.Add stock, cover Instant Pot, and cook on Meat/Stew mode for 45 minutes.
5.Uncover Instant Pot, transfer pork to a platter, shred, and serve.

Nutrition: Calories: 452, Fat: 33.5, Fiber: 0, Carbohydrates: 0, Protein: 35.3

Beef Zucchini Cups

Prep Time: 10 minutes **Cook Time:** 35 minutes
Servings: 4

Ingredients:
2 garlic cloves, peeled and minced
1 teaspoon cumin
1 tablespoon coconut oil
1 pound ground beef
½ cup onion, chopped
1 teaspoon smoked paprika
Salt and ground black pepper, to taste
3 zucchini, sliced in half lengthwise, and insides scooped out
¼ cup fresh cilantro, chopped
½ cup cheddar cheese, shredded
1½ cups tomato paste
Avocado, chopped, for serving
Green onions, chopped, for serving
Tomatoes, cored, and chopped, for serving

Directions:
1.Heat a pan with oil over medium–high heat, add onions, stir, and cook for 2 minutes.
2.Add beef, stir, and brown for a couple of minutes.
3.Add paprika, salt, pepper, cumin, and garlic, stir, and cook for 2 minutes.
4.Place zucchini halves in a baking pan, stuff each with the beef, pour enchilada sauce on top, and sprinkle with cheddar cheese.
5.Bake covered in oven at 350ºF for 20 minutes.
6.Uncover pan, sprinkle with the cilantro, and bake for 5 minutes.
7.Sprinkle with avocado, green onions, and tomatoes on top, divide on plates, and serve.

Nutrition: Calories: 622, Fat: 17.1, Fiber: 16.7, Carbohydrates: 74.6, Protein: 55.4

Beef and Tomato–stuffed Squash

Prep Time: 10 minutes **Cook Time:** 1 hour
Servings: 2

Ingredients:
1 pound spaghetti squash, pricked with a fork
Salt and ground black pepper, to taste
3 garlic cloves, peeled and minced
1 onion, peeled and chopped
1 Portobello mushroom, sliced
28 ounces canned diced tomatoes
1 teaspoon dried oregano
¼ teaspoon cayenne pepper
½ teaspoon dried thyme
1 pound ground beef
1 green bell pepper, seeded and chopped

Directions:
1.Place squash on a lined baking sheet, place in oven at 400ºF, and bake for 40 minutes.
2.Cut in half, set aside to cool, remove seeds, and leave aside.
3.Heat a pan over medium–high heat, add meat, garlic, onion, mushroom, stir, and cook until meat browns.
4.Add salt, pepper, thyme, oregano, cayenne, tomatoes, green pepper, stir, and cook for 10 minutes.
5.Stuff squash halves with beef mixture, place in an oven at 400º and bake for 10 minutes.
6.Divide between 2 plates and serve.

Nutrition: Calories: 616, Fat: 16.6, Fiber: 7.3, Carbohydrates: 43.1, Protein:75.5

Beef Meatball Casserole

Prep Time: 10 minutes **Cook Time:** 50 minutes
Servings: 8

Ingredients:
⅓ cup almond flour
2 eggs
1 pound beef sausage, chopped
1 pound ground beef
Salt and ground black pepper, to taste
1 tablespoons dried parsley
¼ teaspoon red pepper flakes
¼ cup Parmesan cheese, grated
¼ teaspoon onion powder
½ teaspoon garlic powder
¼ teaspoon dried oregano
1 cup ricotta cheese
2 cups tomato paste
2 teaspoons minced garlic
2 teaspoons dried basil
1 teaspoon dried rosemary
1½ cups mozzarella cheese, shredded

Directions:
1.In a bowl, mix sausage with beef, salt, pepper, almond flour, parsley, pepper flakes, onion powder, garlic powder, oregano, Parmesan cheese, eggs, and stir well.
2.Shape meatballs, place on a lined baking sheet, place in an oven at 375ºF, and bake for 15 minutes.
3.Take meatballs out of oven, transfer to a baking dish, and cover with half of the tomato paste, galic, basil, and rosemary.
4.Add ricotta cheese all over and then pour rest of the tomato mixture.
5.Sprinkle mozzarella cheese all over, place dish in the oven at 375ºF and bake for 30 minutes.
6.Let casserole cool before cutting and serving.

Nutrition: Calories: 531, Fat: 33.6, Fiber: 3, Carbohydrates: 17.5, Protein: 40.9

Glazed Beef Meatloaf

Prep Time: 10 minutes **Cook Time:** 1 hour and 10 minutes
Servings: 6

Ingredients:
1 cup white mushrooms, chopped
3 pounds ground beef
2 tablespoons fresh parsley, chopped
2 garlic cloves, peeled and minced
½ cup onion, chopped
¼ cup red bell pepper, seeded and chopped
½ cup almond flour
⅓ cup Parmesan cheese, grated
3 eggs
Salt and ground black pepper, to taste
1 teaspoon balsamic vinegar
For the glaze:
1 tablespoon swerve
2 tablespoons tomato passata
2 cups balsamic vinegar

Directions:
1.In a bowl, mix beef with salt, pepper, mushrooms, garlic, onion, bell pepper, parsley, almond flour, Parmesan cheese, 1 teaspoon vinegar, salt, pepper, eggs, and stir well.
2.Transfer into a loaf pan, and bake in oven at 375ºF for 30 minutes.
3.Heat a small pan over medium heat, add tomato passata, swerve, and 2 cups vinegar, stir well, and cook for 20 minutes.
4.Take meatloaf out of oven, spread the glaze on meatloaf, place in oven at the same temperature and bake for 20 minutes. Let the meatloaf cool, slice, and serve it.

Nutrition: Calories: 606, Fat: 26.4, Fiber: 2, Carbohydrates: 8.3, Protein: 79.8

Beef with Tzatziki

Prep Time: 10 minutes **Cook Time:** 15 minutes
Servings: 6

Ingredients:
¼ cup almond milk
17 ounces ground beef
1 onion, peeled, and grated
5 oz cauliflower rice
1 egg, whisked
¼ cup fresh parsley, chopped
Salt and ground black pepper, to taste
2 garlic cloves, peeled and minced
¼ cup fresh mint, chopped
2, and ½ teaspoons dried oregano
¼ cup olive oil
7 ounces cherry tomatoes, cut in half
1 cucumber, sliced thin
1 cup baby spinach
1½ tablespoons lemon juice
7 ounces jarred tzatziki

Directions:
1.Put cauliflower rice in a bowl, add milk, and set aside for 3 minutes.
2.Drain, add beef, egg, salt, pepper, oregano, mint, parsley, garlic, onion, and stir well.
3.Shape balls from mixture and place on a working surface.
4.Heat a pan with half of the oil over medium–high heat, add meatballs, cook them for 8 minutes flipping them from time to time, and transfer them to a tray.
5.In a salad bowl, mix spinach with cucumber and tomato.
6.Add meatballs, remaining oil, and some salt, pepper and lemon juice. Add tzatziki, toss to coat, and serve.

Nutrition: Calories: 322, Fat: 18.6, Fiber: 1.7, Carbohydrates: 9.9, Protein: 29.2

Meatballs with Mushroom Sauce

Prep Time: 10 minutes **Cook Time:** 25 minutes
Servings: 6

Ingredients:
2 pounds ground beef
Salt and ground black pepper, to taste
½ teaspoon garlic powder
1 tablespoon coconut aminos
¼ cup beef stock
¾ cup almond flour
1 tablespoon fresh parsley, chopped
1 tablespoon dried onion flakes
For the sauce:
1 cup onion, chopped
2 cups mushrooms, sliced
2 tablespoons bacon fat
2 tablespoons butter
½ teaspoon coconut aminos
¼ cup sour cream
½ cup beef stock
Salt and ground black pepper, to taste

Directions:
1.In a bowl, mix beef with salt, pepper, garlic powder, 1 tablespoon coconut aminos, ¼ cup beef stock, almond flour, parsley, and onion flakes, stir well, shape 6 patties, place them on a baking sheet, place in an oven at 375ºF and bake for 18 minutes.
2.Heat a pan with butter, and bacon fat over medium heat, add mushrooms, stir, and cook for 4 minutes.
3.Add onions, stir, and cook for 4 minutes. Add ½ teaspoon coconut aminos, sour cream, and ½ cup beef stock, stir well, and bring to a simmer.
4.Take heat, add salt, pepper, and stir well.
5.Divide the beef patties on plates and serve with mushroom sauce on top.

Nutrition: Calories: 452, Fat: 23.5, Fiber: 1.3, Carbohydrates: 4.9, Protein: 53.2

Zucchini Noodles and Beef

Prep Time: 10 minutes **Cook Time:** 20 minutes
Servings: 5

Ingredients:
1 pound ground beef
1 onion, peeled and chopped
2 garlic cloves, peeled and minced
14 ounces canned diced tomatoes
1 tablespoon dried rosemary
1 tablespoon dried sage
1 tablespoon dried oregano
1 tablespoon dried basil
1 tablespoon dried marjoram
Salt and ground black pepper, to taste
2 zucchini, cut with a spiralizer

Directions:
1.Heat a pan over medium heat, add garlic and onion, stir, and brown for a couple of minutes.
2.Add beef, stir, and cook for 6 minutes. Add tomatoes, salt, pepper, rosemary, sage, oregano, marjoram, basil, stir, and simmer for 15 minutes.
3.Divide zucchini noodles into bowls, add beef mixture, and serve.

Nutrition: Calories: 206, Fat: 6, Fiber: 2.3, Carbohydrates: 8.2, Protein: 29.5

Beef Chili

Prep Time: 10 minutes **Cook Time:** 8 hours
Servings: 4

Ingredients:
1 onion, peeled and chopped
2½ pounds ground beef
15 ounces canned tomatoes, and green chilies, chopped
6 ounces tomato paste
½ cup pickled jalapeños, chopped
4 tablespoons garlic, minced
3 celery stalks, chopped
2 tablespoons coconut aminos
4 tablespoons chili powder
Salt and ground black pepper, to taste
A pinch of cayenne pepper
2 tablespoons cumin
1 teaspoon onion powder
1 teaspoon garlic powder
1 bay leaf
1 teaspoon dried oregano

Directions:
1.Heat a pan over medium–high heat, add half of onion, beef, half of the garlic, salt, and pepper, stir, and cook until meat browns.
2.Transfer to a slow cooker, add rest of the onion and garlic, plus jalapeños, celery, tomatoes, chilies, tomato paste, canned tomatoes, coconut aminos, chili powder, salt, pepper, cumin, garlic powder, onion powder, oregano, and bay leaf, stir, cover, and cook on low for 8 hours. Divide into bowls and serve.

Nutrition: Calories: 626, Fat: 19.3, Fiber: 4, Carbohydrates: 19.7, Protein: 89.7

Beef Goulash

Prep Time: 10 minutes **Cook Time:** 20 minutes
Servings: 5

Ingredients:
2 ounces bell pepper, seeded and chopped
1½ pounds ground beef
Salt and ground black pepper, to taste
2 cups cauliflower florets
¼ cup onion, peeled and chopped
14 ounces canned diced tomatoes, and
¼ teaspoon garlic powder
1 tablespoon tomato paste
14 ounces water

Directions:
1.Heat a pan over medium heat, add beef, stir, and brown for 5 minutes.
2.Add onion and bell pepper, stir, and cook for 4 minutes. Add cauliflower, tomatoes, water, stir, bring to a simmer, cover pan, and cook for 5 minutes.
3.Add tomato paste, garlic powder, salt, and pepper, stir, take off heat, divide into bowls, and serve.

Nutrition: Calories: 972, Fat: 31.4, Fiber: 2.9, Carbohydrates: 10.1, Protein: 153.6

Beef and Sauerkraut Soup

Prep Time: 10 minutes **Cook Time:** 1 hour and 20 minutes **Servings:** 8

Ingredients:
3 teaspoons olive oil
1 pound ground beef
14 ounces beef stock
2 cups chicken stock
14 ounces canned tomatoes, and juice
1 tablespoon stevia
14 ounces sauerkraut, chopped
1 tablespoon gluten–free Worcestershire sauce
4 bay leaves
Salt and ground black pepper, to taste
3 tablespoons fresh parsley, chopped
1 onion, peeled and chopped
1 teaspoon dried sage
1 tablespoon garlic, minced
2 cups water

Directions:
1.Heat a pan with 1 teaspoon oil over medium heat, add beef, stir, and brown for 10 minutes.
2.In a pot, mix chicken, beef stock, sauerkraut, stevia, canned tomatoes, Worcestershire sauce, parsley, sage, and bay leaves, stir, and bring to a simmer over medium heat.
3.Add beef to soup, stir, and continue simmering.
4.Heat the same pan with remaining oil over medium heat, add onions, stir, and cook for 2 minutes. Add garlic, stir, cook for 1 minute, and add to the soup.
5.Reduce heat to soup, and simmer it for 1 hour.
6.Add salt, pepper, water, stir, and cook for 15 minutes. Divide into bowls and serve.

Nutrition: Calories: 152, Fat: 1.7, Fiber: 2.5, Carbohydrates: 6, Protein: 19

Jamaican Beef Pies

Prep Time: 10 minutes **Cook Time:** 35 minutes **Servings:** 12

Ingredients:
3 garlic cloves, peeled and minced
½ pound ground beef
½ pound ground pork
½ cup water
1 small onion, peeled and chopped
2 habanero peppers, chopped
2 teaspoons cumin
½ teaspoon turmeric
Salt and ground black pepper, to taste
1 teaspoon garlic powder
¼ teaspoon stevia powder
2 tablespoons butter
For the crust:
4 tablespoons butter, melted
6 ounces cream cheese
A pinch of salt
1 teaspoon turmeric
¼ teaspoon stevia
½ teaspoon baking powder
1½ cups flax meal
2 tablespoons water
½ cup coconut flour

Directions:
1.In a blender, mix onion with habaneros, garlic, and ½ cup water. Heat a pan over medium heat, add pork and beef, stir, and cook for 3 minutes.
2.Add onions mixture, stir, and cook for 2 minutes. Add garlic, onion, curry powder, ½ teaspoon turmeric, salt, pepper, stevia powder, and garlic powder, stir well, and cook for 3 minutes.
3.Add 2 tablespoons butter, stir until it melts, and take off heat. In a bowl, mix 1 teaspoon turmeric, with ¼ teaspoon stevia, baking powder, flax meal, and coconut flour, and stir.
4.In a separate bowl, mix 4 tablespoons butter with 2 tablespoons water and cream cheese, and stir.
5.Combine the 2 mixtures, and mix until you obtain a dough. Shape 12 balls from this mixture, place them on a parchment paper, and roll each into a circle.
6.Divide beef and pork mix on one half of the dough circles, cover with other half, seal edges, and arrange them all on a lined baking sheet.
7.Bake pies in the oven at 350ºF for 25 minutes. Serve warm.

Nutrition: Calories: 198, Fat: 13.6, Fiber: 2.6, Carbohydrates: 5.7, Protein: 13

Ground Beef Casserole

Prep Time: 10 minutes **Cook Time:** 35 minutes **Servings:** 6

Ingredients:
2 teaspoons onion flakes
1 tablespoon gluten–free Worcestershire sauce
2 pounds ground beef
2 garlic cloves, peeled and minced
Salt and ground black pepper, to taste
1 cup mozzarella cheese, shredded
2 cups cheddar cheese, shredded
½ cup keto mayonnaise
2 tablespoons sesame seeds, toasted
20 dill pickle slices
1 romaine lettuce head, torn

Directions:
1.Heat a pan over medium heat, add beef, onion flakes, Worcestershire sauce, salt, pepper, and garlic, stir, and cook for 5 minutes.
2.Transfer to a baking dish, add 1 cup cheddar cheese, mozzarella cheese, and half of mayonnaise. Stir and spread evenly.
3.Arrange pickle slices on top, sprinkle remaining cheddar and sesame seeds, place in an oven at 350ºF and bake for 20 minutes.
4.Turn oven to broil and broil casserole for 5 minutes.
5.Divide lettuce on plates, top with a beef casserole, and remaining mayonnaise.

Nutrition: Calories: 577, Fat: 36.1, Fiber: 1, Carbohydrates: 4.8, Protein: 57.6

Beef and Eggplant Casserole

Prep Time: 30 minutes **Cook Time:** 4 hours **Servings:** 12

Ingredients:
1 tablespoon olive oil
2 pounds ground beef
2 cups eggplant, chopped
Salt and ground black pepper, to taste
2 teaspoons mustard
2 teaspoons gluten–free Worcestershire sauce
28 ounces canned diced tomatoes
2 cups mozzarella cheese, grated
16 ounces tomato sauce
2 tablespoons fresh parsley, chopped
1 teaspoon dried oregano

Directions:
1.Season eggplant pieces with salt and pepper, set aside for 30 minutes, squeeze water a bit, put them into a bowl, add the olive oil, and toss them to coat.
2.In another bowl, mix beef with salt, pepper, mustard, Worcestershire sauce, and stir well. Press them on the bottom of a slow cooker.
3.Add eggplant and spread the pieces out.
4.Add tomatoes, tomato sauce, parsley, oregano, and mozzarella cheese.
5.Cover slow cooker and cook on low for 4 hours. Divide the casserole on plates and serve hot.

Nutrition: Calories: 191, Fat: 7.1, Fiber: 1.9, Carbohydrates: 6.1, Protein: 25.6

Roasted Pork Belly

Prep Time: 10 minutes **Cook Time:** 1 hour and 30 minutes **Servings:** 6

Ingredients:
2 tablespoons stevia
1 tablespoon lemon juice
1 quart water
17 ounces chayote squash, cored, and cut into wedges
2 pounds pork belly, scored
Salt and ground black pepper, to taste
A drizzle of olive oil

Directions:
1.In a blender, mix water with squash, lemon juice, and stevia, and pulse well.
2.Put pork belly in a steamer tray and steam for 1 hour.
3.Transfer pork belly to a baking sheet, rub with drizzle of oil, season with salt and pepper, and pour squash sauce over it.
4.Place in oven at 425ºF for 30 minutes.
5.Slice pork roast, divide on plates, and serve.

Nutrition: Calories: 723, Fat: 40.7, Fiber: 0.9, Carbohydrates: 5.9, Protein: 70.6

Pork Chops with Mushrooms

Prep Time: 10 minutes **Cook Time:** 40 minutes
Servings: 3

Ingredients:
8 ounces mushrooms, sliced
1 teaspoon garlic powder
1 onion, peeled and chopped
1 cup sugar-free mayonnaise
3 pork chops, boneless
1 teaspoon ground nutmeg
1 tablespoon balsamic vinegar
½ cup coconut oil

Directions:
1.Heat a pan with oil over medium heat, add mushrooms and onions, stir, and cook for 4 minutes.
2.Add pork chops, season with nutmeg, and garlic powder, and brown on both sides. Place pan in the oven at 350ºF and bake for 30 minutes.
3.Transfer pork chops to plates and keep warm.
4.Heat the pan over medium heat, add vinegar and mayonnaise over mushrooms mixture, stir well, and take off heat.
5.Drizzle sauce over pork chops and serve.

Nutrition: Calories: 913, Fat: 82.9, Fiber: 1.8, Carbohydrates: 7, Protein: 21.7

Cranberry Pork Roast

Prep Time: 10 minutes **Cook Time:** 8 hours
Servings: 4

Ingredients:
1 tablespoon coconut flour
Salt and ground black pepper, to taste
1½ pounds pork loin
A pinch of dry mustard
½ teaspoon ginger
2 tablespoons erythritol
½ cup cranberries
2 garlic cloves, peeled and minced
½ lemon sliced
¼ cup water

Directions:
1.In a bowl, mix ginger with mustard, salt, pepper, and flour, and stir.
2.Add roast, toss to coat, and transfer meat to a slow cooker.
3.Add erythritol, cranberries, garlic, water, and lemon slices.
4.Cover slow cooker and cook on low for 8 hours.
5.Divide on plates, drizzle pan juices on top, and serve.

Nutrition: Calories: 1523, Fat: 86.9, Fiber: 0.9, Carbohydrates: 7.7, Protein: 170.7

Lemon and Garlic Pork

Prep Time: 10 minutes **Cook Time:** 30 minutes
Servings: 4

Ingredients:
3 tablespoons butter
4 pork steaks, bone–in
1 cup chicken stock
Salt and ground black pepper, to taste
A pinch of lemon pepper
3 tablespoons coconut oil
6 garlic cloves, peeled and minced
2 tablespoons fresh parsley, chopped
8 ounces mushrooms, chopped
1 lemon, sliced

Directions:
1.Heat a pan with 2 tablespoons butter and 2 tablespoons oil over medium–high heat, add pork steaks, season with salt and pepper, cook until brown on both sides, and transfer to a plate.
2.Return pan to medium heat, add rest of the butter, oil, and half of the stock. Stir well, and cook for 1 minute.
3.Add mushrooms and garlic, stir, and cook for 4 minutes. Add lemon slices, rest of the stock, salt, pepper, and lemon pepper, stir, and cook everything for 5 minutes.
4.Return pork steaks to pan and cook everything for 10 minutes.
5.Divide steaks and sauce on plates and serve.

Nutrition: Calories: 665, Fat: 49.2, Fiber: 1.1, Carbohydrates: 5, Protein: 47.6

Juicy Pork Chops

Prep Time: 10 minutes **Cook Time:** 45 minutes
Servings: 4

Ingredients:
2 onions, peeled and chopped
6 bacon slices, chopped
½ cup chicken stock
Salt and ground black pepper, to taste
4 pork chops

Directions:
1.Heat a pan over medium heat, add bacon, stir, cook until crispy and transfer to a bowl.
2.Return pan to medium heat, add onions and some salt and pepper, stir, cover, cook for 15 minutes, and transfer to the same bowl with bacon.
3.Return to heat, increase to medium–high, add pork chops, season with salt and pepper, brown for 3 minutes on one side, flip, reduce heat to medium, and cook for 7 minutes.
4.Add stock, stir, and cook for 2 minutes.
5.Return bacon and onions to the pan, stir, cook for 1 minute, divide on plates, and serve.

Nutrition: Calories: 433, Fat: 31.9, Fiber: 1.2, Carbohydrates: 5.6, Protein: 29.2

Stuffed Pork

Prep Time: 10 minutes **Cook Time:** 30 minutes
Servings: 4

Ingredients:
Zest of 2 limes
Zest from 1 lemon
Juice from 1 lemon
Juice from 2 limes
4 teaspoons garlic, peeled, and minced
¾ cup olive oil
1 cup fresh cilantro, chopped
1 cup fresh mint, chopped
1 teaspoon dried oregano
Salt and ground black pepper, to taste
2 teaspoons cumin
4 pork loin steaks
2 pickles, chopped
4 ham slices
6 Swiss cheese slices
2 tablespoons mustard

Directions:
1.In a food processor, mix lime zest, lime juice, lemon zest, lemon juice, garlic, oil, cilantro, mint, oregano, cumin, salt, pepper, and blend well.
2.Season steaks with salt and pepper, place them into a bowl, add marinade, toss to coat, and set aside for a couple of hours.
3.Place steaks on a working surface, divide pickles, cheese, mustard, and ham on them, roll, and secure with toothpicks.
4.Heat a pan over medium–high heat, add pork rolls, cook for 2 minutes on each side, and transfer to a baking sheet.
5.Place in oven at 350ºF, and bake for 25 minutes. Divide on plates and serve.

Nutrition: Calories: 1157, Fat: 75.1, Fiber: 4.6, Carbohydrates: 13.5, Protein: 113.2

Mediterranean Pork

Prep Time: 10 minutes **Cook Time:** 35 minutes
Servings: 4

Ingredients:
4 pork chops, bone–in
Salt and ground black pepper, to taste
1 teaspoon dried rosemary
3 garlic cloves, peeled and minced

Directions:
1.Season pork chops with salt and pepper, and place in a roasting pan.
2.Add rosemary and garlic, place in an oven at 425ºF and bake for 10 minutes.
3.Reduce heat to 350ºF and roast for 25 minutes.
4.Slice pork, divide on plates, and drizzle with pan juices all over.

Nutrition: Calories: 259, Fat: 19.9, Fiber: 0.1, Carbohydrates: 0.7, Protein: 18.1

Lemon Pork Chops

Prep Time: 10 minutes **Cook Time:** 15 minutes
Servings: 4

Ingredients:
4 medium pork loin chops
1 teaspoon Dijon mustard
1 tablespoon Worcestershire sauce
1 teaspoon lemon juice
1 tablespoon water
Salt and ground black pepper, to taste
1 teaspoon lemon pepper
1 tablespoon butter
1 tablespoon fresh chives, chopped

Directions:
1.In a bowl, mix water with Worcestershire sauce, mustard, and lemon juice, and whisk.
2.Heat a pan with butter over medium heat, add pork chops, season with salt, pepper, and lemon pepper, cook them for 6 minutes, flip, and cook for 6 more minutes.
3.Transfer pork chops to a platter and keep warm.
4.Heat the pan again, add mustard sauce, and bring to a gentle simmer.
5.Pour over pork, sprinkle with chives, and serve.

Nutrition: Calories: 847, Fat: 66.3, Fiber: 0.1, Carbohydrates: 0.9, Protein: 57.4

Italian Pork Chops

Prep Time: 10 minutes **Cook Time:** 40 minutes
Servings: 4

Ingredients:
4 pork chops
1 tablespoon fresh oregano, chopped
2 garlic cloves, peeled and minced
1 tablespoon canola oil
15 ounces canned diced tomatoes
1 tablespoon tomato paste
Salt and ground black pepper, to taste
¼ cup tomato juice

Directions:
1.Heat a pan with oil over medium–high heat, add pork chops, season with salt and pepper, cook for 3 minutes, flip, cook for 3 minutes, and transfer to a plate.
2.Return pan to medium heat, add garlic, stir, and cook for 10 seconds.
3.Add tomato juice, tomatoes, tomato paste, stir, bring to a boil and reduce heat to medium–low.
4.Add pork chops, stir, cover pan, simmer everything for 30 minutes.
5.Transfer pork chops to plates, add oregano to pan, stir, and cook for 2 minutes.
6.Pour over the pork and serve.

Nutrition: Calories: 318, Fat: 23.8, Fiber: 2, Carbohydrates: 6.8, Protein: 19.4

Spicy Pork Chops

Prep Time: 4 hours and 10 minutes **Cook Time:** 15 minutes **Servings:** 4

Ingredients:
¼ cup lime juice
4 pork rib chops
1 tablespoon coconut oil, melted
2 garlic cloves, peeled and minced
1 tablespoon chili powder
1 teaspoon ground cinnamon
2 teaspoons cumin
Salt and ground black pepper, to taste
½ teaspoon chili powder

Directions:
1.In a bowl, mix lime juice with oil, garlic, cumin, cinnamon, chili powder, salt, pepper, chili powder, and whisk.
2.Add pork chops, toss to coat, and set aside in the refrigerator for 4 hours.
3.Place pork on a preheated grill pan over medium heat, cook for 7 minutes, flip, and cook for 7 minutes. Divide on plates and serve.

Nutrition: Calories: 507, Fat: 32.7, Fiber: 0.1, Carbohydrates: 1.4, Protein: 51.9

Braised Lamb Chops

Prep Time: 10 minutes **Cook Time:** 2 hours and 20 minutes **Servings:** 4

Ingredients:
8 lamb chops
1 teaspoon garlic powder
Salt and ground black pepper, to taste
2 teaspoons fresh mint, crushed
A drizzle of olive oil
1 shallot, peeled and chopped
1 cup white wine
Juice of ½ lemon
1 bay leaf
2 cups beef stock
Fresh parsley, chopped, for serving
For the sauce:
2 cups cranberries
½ teaspoon fresh rosemary, chopped
½ cup swerve
1 teaspoon dried mint
Juice of ½ lemon
1 teaspoon fresh ginger, grated
1 cup water
1 teaspoon harissa paste

Directions:
1.In a bowl, mix lamb chops with salt, pepper, 1 teaspoon garlic powder, 2 teaspoons mint, and rub well.
2.Heat a pan with a drizzle of oil over medium–high heat, add lamb chops, brown on all sides, and transfer to a plate.
3.Heat the same pan again over medium–high heat, add shallots, stir, and cook for 1 minute. Add wine and bay leaf, stir, and cook for 4 minutes.
4.Add 2 cups beef stock, parsley, and juice from ½ lemon, stir, and simmer for 5 minutes. Return lamb, stir, and cook for 10 minutes.
5.Cover pan, and place it in the oven at 350ºF for 2 hours.
6.Heat a pan over medium–high heat, add cranberries, swerve, rosemary, 1 teaspoon mint, juice from ½ lemon, ginger, water, harissa paste, stir, bring to a simmer for 15 minutes.
7.Take lamb chops out of oven, divide them on plates, drizzle cranberry sauce over them, and serve.

Nutrition: Calories: 1148, Fat: 42, Fiber: 2.3, Carbohydrates: 7.6, Protein: 160.9

Italian Pork Rolls

Prep Time: 10 minutes **Cook Time:** 20 minutes **Servings:** 6

Ingredients:
6 prosciutto slices
2 tablespoons fresh parsley, chopped
1 pound pork cutlets, sliced thin
⅓ cup ricotta cheese
1 tablespoon coconut oil
¼ cup onion, chopped
3 garlic cloves, peeled and minced
2 tablespoons Parmesan cheese, grated
15 ounces canned diced tomatoes
⅓ cup chicken stock
Salt and ground black pepper, to taste
½ teaspoon Italian seasoning

Directions:
1.Use a meat pounder to flatten pork pieces.
2.Place prosciutto slices on top of each piece, then divide ricotta cheese, parsley, and Parmesan cheese.
3.Roll each pork piece and secure with a toothpick.
4.Heat a pan with oil over medium heat, add pork rolls, cook until brown on both sides, and transfer to a plate.
5.Heat the pan again over medium heat, add garlic and onion, stir, and cook for 5 minutes.
6.Add stock and cook for 3 minutes.
7.Discard toothpicks from pork rolls and return to the pan.
8.Add tomatoes, Italian seasoning, salt, and pepper, stir, bring to a boil, reduce heat to medium–low, cover pan, and cook for 30 minutes.
9.Divide on plates and serve.

Nutrition: Calories: 256, Fat: 13.9, Fiber: 2.1, Carbohydrates: 15.7, Protein: 17.2

Lamb Curry

Prep Time: 10 minutes **Cook Time:** 4 hours
Servings: 6

Ingredients:
2 tablespoons fresh ginger, grated
2 garlic cloves, peeled and minced
2 teaspoons cardamom
1 onion, peeled and chopped
6 cloves
1 pound lamb meat, cubed
2 teaspoons cumin powder
1 teaspoon garam masala
½ teaspoon chili powder
1 teaspoon turmeric
2 teaspoons coriander
1 pound spinach
14 ounces canned diced tomatoes

Directions:
1.In a slow cooker, mix lamb with spinach, tomatoes, ginger, garlic, onion, cardamom, cloves, cumin, garam masala, chili, turmeric, and coriander, stir, cover, and cook on high for 4 hours.
2.Uncover slow cooker, stir the chili, divide into bowls, and serve.

Nutrition: Calories: 186, Fat: 6.1, Fiber: 3.3, Carbohydrates: 9.1, Protein: 24.3

Lamb Salad

Prep Time: 10 minutes **Cook Time:** 35 minutes
Servings: 4

Ingredients:
1 tablespoon olive oil
3 pounds leg of lamb, bone removed, and leg butterflied
Salt and ground black pepper, to taste
1 teaspoon cumin
A pinch of dried thyme
2 garlic cloves, peeled and minced
For the salad:
4 ounces feta cheese, crumbled
½ cup pecans
2 cups spinach
1½ tablespoons lemon juice
¼ cup olive oil
1 cup fresh mint, chopped

Directions:
1.Rub lamb with salt, pepper, 1 tablespoon oil, thyme, cumin, and minced garlic, place on preheated grill pan over medium–high heat and cook for 40 minutes, flipping once.
2.Spread pecans on a lined baking sheet, place in an oven at 350ºF, and toast for 10 minutes.
3.Transfer grilled lamb to a cutting board, set aside to cool down, and slice.
4.In a salad bowl, mix spinach with 1 cup mint, feta cheese, ¼ cup olive oil, lemon juice, toasted pecans, salt, and pepper, and toss to coat.
5.Add lamb slices on top and serve.

Nutrition: Calories: 931, Fat: 52.5, Fiber: 4.7, Carbohydrates: 8.3, Protein: 103.7

Paprika Lamb Chops

Prep Time: 10 minutes **Cook Time:** 15 minutes
Servings: 4

Ingredients:
2 lamb racks, cut into chops
Salt and ground black pepper, to taste
3 tablespoons paprika
¾ cup cumin powder
1 teaspoon chili powder

Directions:
1.In a bowl, mix paprika with cumin, chili, salt, pepper, and stir.
2.Add lamb chops and rub them well.
3.Heat a grill over medium temperature, add lamb chops, cook for 5 minutes, flip, and cook for 5 minutes.
4.Flip again, cook for 2 minutes, and then for 2 minutes on the other side again.

Nutrition: Calories: 392, Fat: 17, Fiber: 4.1, Carbohydrates: 11.6, Protein: 50.1

Lamb with Mustard Sauce

Prep Time: 10 minutes **Cook Time:** 20 minutes **Servings:** 4

Ingredients:

2 tablespoons olive oil
1 tablespoon fresh rosemary, chopped
2 garlic cloves, peeled and minced
1½ pounds lamb chops
Salt and ground black pepper, to taste
1 tablespoon shallot, peeled and chopped
⅔ cup heavy cream
½ cup beef stock
1 tablespoon mustard
2 teaspoons gluten–free Worcestershire sauce
2 teaspoons lemon juice
1 teaspoon erythritol
2 tablespoons butter
A sprig of rosemary
A sprig of thyme

Directions:

1.In a bowl, mix 1 tablespoon oil with garlic, salt, pepper, rosemary, and whisk.
2.Add lamb chops, toss to coat, and set aside for a few minutes.
3.Heat a pan with rest of the oil over medium–high heat, add lamb chops, reduce heat to medium, cook them for 7 minutes, flip, cook them for 7 minutes, transfer to a plate and keep them warm.
4.Return pan to medium heat, add shallots, stir, and cook for 3 minutes.
5.Add stock, stir, and cook for 1 minute.
6.Add Worcestershire sauce, mustard, erythritol, cream, rosemary, thyme, stir, and cook for 8 minutes.
7.Add lemon juice, salt, pepper, and butter, discard the rosemary and thyme, stir well, and take off the heat.
8.Divide lamb chops on plates, drizzle the sauce over them, and serve.

Nutrition: Calories: 1363, Fat: 66.9, Fiber: 0.8, Carbohydrates: 4.6 Protein: 176.9

Lamb Casserole

Prep Time: 10 minutes **Cook Time:** 1 hour and 40 minutes **Servings:** 2

Ingredients:

2 garlic cloves, peeled and minced
1 onion, peeled and chopped
1 tablespoon olive oil
1 celery stalk, chopped
10 ounces lamb fillet, cut into medium–sized pieces
Salt and ground black pepper, to taste
1¼ cups lamb stock
5 oz butternut squash, peeled and chopped
½ tablespoon fresh rosemary, chopped
1 leek, chopped
½ oz finely shredded mint leaves
1 teaspoon stevia
1 tablespoon tomato puree
½ cauliflower, separated into florets
½ celeriac, chopped
2 tablespoons butter

Directions:

1.Heat a pot with oil over medium heat, add garlic, onion, celery, stir, and cook for 5 minutes.
2.Add lamb pieces, stir, and cook for 3 minutes.
3.Add squash, leek, rosemary, stock, tomato puree, mint leaves, stevia, stir, bring to a boil, cover, and cook for 1 hour and 30 minutes.
4.Heat a pot with water over medium heat, add celeriac, cover, and simmer for 10 minutes.
5.Add cauliflower florets, cook for 15 minutes, drain everything, and mix with salt, pepper, and butter.
6.Mash using a potato masher, and divide the mash on plates.
7.Add lamb and vegetables mixture on top and serve.

Nutrition: Calories: 1241, Fat: 29.6, Fiber: 6.9, Carbohydrates: 57.3, Protein: 154.4

Lamb Stew

Prep Time: 10 minutes **Cook Time:** 3 hours
Servings: 4

Ingredients:
1 onion, peeled and chopped
7 oz butternut squash, peeled and chopped
2 pounds lamb, cubed
1 tomato, cored and chopped
1 garlic clove, peeled and minced
2 tablespoons butter
1 cup beef stock
1 cup white wine
Salt and ground black pepper, to taste
2 rosemary sprigs
1 teaspoon fresh thyme, chopped

Directions:
1.Heat a Dutch oven over medium–high heat, add oil, and heat up.
2.Add lamb, salt, and pepper, brown on all sides, and transfer to a plate.
3.Add onion to Dutch oven and cook for 2 minutes. Add squash, tomato, garlic, butter, stick, wine, salt, pepper, rosemary, thyme, stir, and cook for a couple of minutes.
4.Return lamb to Dutch oven, stir, reduce heat to medium–low, cover, and cook for 4 hours.
5.Discard rosemary sprigs, add more salt and pepper, stir, divide into bowls, and serve.

Nutrition: Calories: 564, Fat: 22.6, Fiber: 1.9, Carbohydrates: 11, Protein: 65.5

Slow–cooked Leg of Lamb

Prep Time: 10 minutes **Cook Time:** 8 hours
Servings: 6

Ingredients:
2 pounds lamb leg
Salt and ground black pepper, to taste
1 tablespoon maple extract
2 tablespoons mustard
¼ cup olive oil
4 thyme sprigs
6 mint leaves
1 teaspoon garlic, minced
A pinch of dried rosemary

Directions:
1.Put oil in a slow cooker. Add lamb, salt, pepper, maple extract, mustard, rosemary, garlic, rub well, cover, and cook on low for 7 hours.
2.Add mint and thyme, and cook for 1 hour.
3.Rest the lamb before slicing and serving with pan juices on top.

Nutrition: Calories: 390, Fat: 20.3, Fiber: 1.7, Carbohydrates: 3.6, Protein: 46

Lavender Lamb Chops

Prep Time: 10 minutes **Cook Time:** 25 minutes
Servings: 4

Ingredients:
2 tablespoons rosemary, chopped
1½ pounds lamb chops
Salt and ground black pepper, to taste
1 tablespoon fresh lavender, chopped
2 garlic cloves, peeled and minced
3 lemons, cut in half
2 small pieces of orange peel
A drizzle of olive oil

Directions:
1.In a bowl, mix lamb chops with salt, pepper, rosemary, lavender, garlic, orange peel, toss to coat, and set aside for a couple of hours.
2.Grease a kitchen grill with butter, heat over medium–high heat, place lamb chops, cook for 3 minutes, flip, squeeze 1 lemon half over them, cook for 3 minutes, flip them again, cook them for 2 minutes and squeeze another lemon half over them.
3.Place lamb chops on a plate and keep them warm for now.
4.Add remaining lemon half on preheated grill, cook them for 3 minutes, flip, and cook for another 3 minutes.
5.Divide lamb chops on plates, add lemon halves on the side, drizzle some olive oil, and serve.

Nutrition: Calories: 1171, Fat: 46, Fiber: 0.9, Carbohydrates: 2.3, Protein: 175.4

Lamb with Lemon Dressing

Prep Time: 10 minutes **Cook Time:** 4 hours
Servings: 4

Ingredients:
2 lamb shanks
Salt and ground black pepper, to taste
1 garlic head, peeled
4 tablespoons olive oil
Juice of ½ lemon
Zest from ½ lemon
½ teaspoon dried oregano

Directions:
1.In a slow cooker, mix lamb with salt and pepper.
2.Add garlic, cover, and cook on high for 4 hours. In a bowl, mix lemon juice with lemon zest, some salt and pepper, olive oil, oregano, and whisk.
3.Uncover slow cooker, shred the lamb, discard bone and divide on plates.
4.Drizzle lemon dressing all over and serve.

Nutrition: Calories: 434, Fat: 26.1, Fiber: 0.7, Carbohydrates: 2.8, Protein: 46.3

Moroccan Lamb

Prep Time: 10 minutes **Cook Time:** 15 minutes
Servings: 4

Ingredients:
2 teaspoons paprika
2 garlic cloves, peeled and minced
2 teaspoons dried oregano
2 tablespoons sumac
12 lamb cutlets
¼ cup olive oil
2 tablespoons water
2 teaspoons cumin
10 oz butternut squash peeled, and sliced
¼ cup fresh parsley, chopped
2 teaspoons harissa
1 tablespoon red wine vinegar
Salt and ground black pepper, to taste
2 tablespoons black olives, pitted and sliced
6 radishes, sliced thin

Directions:
1.In a bowl, mix cutlets with paprika, garlic, oregano, sumac, salt, pepper, half of the oil and water, and rub well.
2.Put squash in a pot, add water to cover, bring to a boil over medium–high heat, cook for 2 minutes drain, and put in a salad bowl. Add olives and radishes to squahs.
3.In another bowl, mix harissa with remaining oil, parsley, cumin, vinegar, a splash of water, and stir well.
4.Add to squash mixture, season with salt and pepper, and toss to coat.
5.Heat a kitchen grill over medium–high heat, add lamb cutlets, grill them for 3 minutes on each side, and divide them on plates.
6.Add squash salad on the side and serve.

Nutrition: Calories: 737, Fat: 37.7, Fiber: 0.5, Carbohydrates: 2.2, Protein: 92.4

Lamb Riblets and Mint Pesto

Prep Time: 1 hour **Cook Time:** 2 hours
Servings: 4

Ingredients:
1 cup parsley
1 cup mint
1½onions, peeled and chopped
⅓ cup pistachios
1 teaspoon lemon zest
5 tablespoons avocado oil
Salt, to taste
2 pounds lamb riblets
5 garlic cloves, peeled and minced
Juice from 1 lemon

Directions:
1.In a food processor, mix parsley with mint, 1 onion, pistachios, lemon zest, salt, avocado oil, and blend well.
2.Rub lamb with this mixture, place in a bowl, cover, and leave in the refrigerator for 1 hour.
3.Transfer lamb to a baking dish, add garlic, and ½ onion to the dish, drizzle with lemon juice, and bake in oven at 250ºF for 2 hours.
4.Divide on plates and serve.

Nutrition: Calories: 870, Fat: 47.4, Fiber: 6.7, Carbohydrates: 20.7, Protein: 87.5

Lamb with Fennel and Prunes

Prep Time: 10 minutes **Cook Time:** 40 minutes
Servings: 4

Ingredients:
12 ounces lamb racks
2 fennel bulbs, sliced
Salt and ground black pepper, to taste
2 tablespoons olive oil
4 prunes, cut in half
⅛ cup apple cider vinegar
1 tablespoon swerve

Directions:
1.In a bowl, mix fennel with prunes, vinegar, swerve, and oil, toss to coat well, and transfer to a baking dish.
2.Season with salt and pepper, place in an oven at 400ºF and bake for 15 minutes.
3.Season lamb with salt and pepper, place into a heated pan over medium–high heat and cook for a couple of minutes.
4.Add lamb to the baking dish with fennel and prunes, place in oven, and bake for 20 minutes.
5.Divide everything on plates and serve.

Nutrition: Calories: 375, Fat: 13.7, Fiber: 7.2, Carbohydrates: 40.7, Protein: 26.4

Baked Veal and Cabbage

Prep Time: 10 minutes **Cook Time:** 40 minutes
Servings: 4

Ingredients:
17 ounces veal, cut into cubes
1 cabbage head, shredded
Salt and ground black pepper, to taste
3. 4 ounces ham, chopped
1 onion, peeled and chopped
2 garlic cloves, peeled and minced
1 tablespoon butter
½ cup Parmesan cheese, grated
½ cup sour cream

Directions:
1.Heat a pot with butter over medium–high heat, add onion, stir, and cook for 2 minutes. Add garlic, stir, and cook for 1 minute.
2.Add ham and veal, stir and cook until slightly browned.
3.Add cabbage, stir and cook until it softens, and meat is tender.
4.Add cream, salt, pepper, cheese, stir gently, place in an oven at 350ºF and bake for 20 minutes.
5.Divide on plates and serve.

Nutrition: Calories: 535, Fat: 28.5, Fiber: 6.2, Carbohydrates: 18.4, Protein: 51.6

Slow–roasted Beef

Prep Time: 10 minutes **Cook Time:** 8 hours
Servings: 8

Ingredients:
5 pounds beef joint
Salt and ground black pepper, to taste
½ teaspoon celery salt
2 teaspoons chili powder
1 tablespoon avocado oil
1 tablespoon sweet paprika
A pinch of cayenne pepper
½ teaspoon garlic powder
½ cup beef stock
1 tablespoon garlic, minced
¼ teaspoon dry mustard

Directions:
1.Heat a pan with oil over medium–high heat, add beef and brown it on all sides.
2.In a bowl, mix paprika with chili powder, celery salt, salt, pepper, cayenne, garlic powder, dry mustard, and stir.
3.Add roast, rub well, and transfer it to a slow cooker.
4.Add beef stock and garlic over roast and cook on low for 8 hours.
5.Transfer beef to a cutting board, leave it to cool, slice, and divide on plates.
6.Strain the juices from the pot, drizzle over the meat, and serve.

Nutrition: Calories: 430, Fat: 9.9, Fiber: 0.4, Carbohydrates: 4.1, Protein: 76

Beef Bourguignon

Prep Time: 3 hours and 10 minutes **Cook Time:** 5 hours and 15 minutes
Servings: 8

Ingredients:
3 tablespoons olive oil
2 tablespoons onion, peeled and chopped
1 tablespoon dried parsley flakes
1½ cups red wine
1 teaspoon dried thyme
Salt and ground black pepper, to taste
1 bay leaf
⅓ cup almond flour
4 pounds beef, cubed
24 small white onions
8 bacon slices, chopped
2 garlic cloves, peeled and minced
1 pound mushrooms, chopped

Directions:
1.In a bowl, mix wine with olive oil, minced onion, thyme, parsley, salt, pepper, bay leaf, and whisk.
2.Add beef cubes, stir, and set aside for 3 hours.
3.Drain meat, and reserve 1 cup of marinade. Add flour over meat, and toss to coat.
4.Heat a pan over medium–high heat, add bacon, stir and cook until slightly browned.
5.Add onions, stir, and cook for 3 minutes. Add garlic, stir, cook for 1 minute, and transfer everything to a slow cooker. Add meat to slow cooker and stir.
6.Heat the pan with bacon fat over medium–high heat, add mushrooms and onions, stir, and sauté for a couple of minutes.
7.Add to slow cooker as well with reserved marinade, some salt and pepper, cover, and cook on high for 5 hours. Divide on plates and serve.

Nutrition: Calories: 734, Fat: 27.5, Fiber: 1.6, Carbohydrates: 10.8, Protein: 78.3

Beef Stew

Prep Time: 10 minutes **Cook Time:** 4 hours and 10 minutes
Servings: 4

Ingredients:
8 ounces pancetta, chopped
4 pounds beef, cubed
4 garlic cloves, peeled and minced
2 brown onions, peeled and chopped
2 tablespoons olive oil
4 tablespoons red vinegar
4 cups beef stock
2 tablespoons tomato paste
2 cinnamon sticks
3 lemon peel strips
½ cup fresh parsley, chopped
4 thyme sprigs
2 tablespoons butter
Salt and ground black pepper, to taste

Directions:
1.Heat a pan with oil over medium–high heat, add pancetta, onion, garlic, stir, and cook for 5 minutes.
2.Add beef, stir, and cook until it browns.
3.Add the vinegar, salt, pepper, stock, tomato paste, cinnamon, lemon peel, thyme, butter, stir, cook for 3 minutes, and transfer everything to a slow cooker.
4.Cover and cook on high for 4 hours.
5.Discard cinnamon, lemon peel, and thyme, add the parsley, stir, and divide into bowls. Serve hot.

Nutrition: Calories: 1318, Fat: 65.5, Fiber: 2.2, Carbohydrates: 9.7, Protein: 162.9

Pork Stew

Prep Time: 10 minutes **Cook Time:** 1 hour and 20 minutes **Servings:** 12

Ingredients:
2 tablespoons coconut oil
4 pounds pork, cubed
Salt and ground black pepper, to taste
2 tablespoons butter
3 garlic cloves, peeled and minced
¾ cup beef stock
¾ cup apple cider vinegar
5 oz butternut squash, peeled and chopped
1 cabbage head, shredded
½ cup green onion, chopped
1 cup heavy cream

Directions:
1.Heat a pan with butter and oil over medium–high heat, add pork and brown it for a few minutes on each side.
2.Add vinegar and stock, stir well, and bring to a simmer.
3.Add cabbage, garlic, salt, and pepper, stir, cover, and cook for 1 hour.
4.Add squash and green onions, stir, and cook for 15 minutes.
5.Add heavy cream, stir for 1 minute, divide on plates, and serve.

Nutrition: Calories: 314, Fat: 13.3, Fiber: 1.9, Carbohydrates: 5.8, Protein: 41

Sausage Stew

Prep Time: 10 minutes **Cook Time:** 20 minutes **Servings:** 9

Ingredients:
1 pound smoked sausage, sliced
1 green bell pepper, seeded and chopped
2 onions, peeled and chopped
Salt and ground black pepper, to taste
1 cup fresh parsley, chopped
8 green onions, chopped
¼ cup avocado oil
1 cup beef stock
6 garlic cloves
28 ounces canned diced tomatoes
16 ounces okra, trimmed and sliced
8 ounces tomato passata
2 tablespoons coconut aminos
1 tablespoon cayenne pepper powder

Directions:
1.Heat a pot with oil over medium–high heat, add sausages, stir, and cook for 2 minutes.
2.Add onion, bell pepper, green onions, parsley, salt, and pepper, stir, and cook for 2 minutes.
3.Add stock, garlic, tomatoes, okra, tomato passata, coconut aminos, cayenne pepper, stir, bring to a simmer, and cook for 15 minutes.
4.Add more salt, pepper, stir, divide into bowls, and serve.

Nutrition: Calories: 253, Fat: 15.7, Fiber: 4.4, Carbohydrates: 15.2, Protein: 13.3

Burgundy Beef Stew

Prep Time: 10 minutes **Cook Time:** 3 hours **Servings:** 7

Ingredients:
2 pounds beef chuck roast, cubed
15 ounces canned diced tomatoes
10 oz butternut squash, peeled and chopped
Salt and ground black pepper, to taste
½ pounds mushrooms, sliced
2 celery stalks, chopped
2 onions, peeled and chopped
1 cup beef stock
1 tablespoon fresh thyme, chopped
½ teaspoon dry mustard
3 tablespoons almond flour
1 cup water

Directions:
1.Heat an ovenproof pot over medium–high heat, add beef cubes, stir, and brown for a couple of minutes on each side.
2.Add tomatoes, mushrooms, onions, squash, celery, salt, pepper mustard, stock, thyme, and stir. In a bowl, mix water with flour and stir well.
3.Add to pot, stir well, place in oven, and bake at 325ºF for 3 hours.
4.Stir every 30 minutes. Divide into bowls and serve.

Nutrition: Calories: 547, Fat: 38.5, Fiber: 3.2, Carbohydrates: 12.4, Protein: 37.6

Cuban Beef Stew

Prep Time: 10 minutes **Cook Time:** 6 hours
Servings: 8

Ingredients:
2 onions, peeled and chopped
2 tablespoons avocado oil
2 pounds beef roast, cubed
2 green bell peppers, seeded and chopped
1 habanero pepper, chopped
4 jalapeños, chopped
14 ounces canned diced tomatoes
2 tablespoons fresh cilantro, chopped
6 garlic cloves, peeled and minced
½ cup water
Salt and ground black pepper, to taste
1½ teaspoons cumin
4 teaspoons bouillon granules
½ cup black olives, pitted and chopped
1 teaspoon dried oregano

Directions:
1.Heat a pan with oil over medium–high heat, add beef, brown it on all sides and transfer to a slow cooker.
2.Add green bell peppers, onions, jalapeños, habanero pepper, tomatoes, garlic, water, bouillon, cilantro, oregano, cumin, salt, pepper, and stir.
3.Cover slow cooker, and cook on low for 6 hours.
4.Add olives, stir, divide into bowls, and serve.

Nutrition: Calories: 267, Fat: 9, Fiber: 2.5, Carbohydrates: 9.7, Protein: 36

Ham Stew

Prep Time: 10 minutes **Cook Time:** 4 hours
Servings: 6

Ingredients:
8 ounces cheddar cheese, grated
14 ounces chicken stock
½ teaspoon garlic powder
½ teaspoon onion powder
Salt and ground black pepper, to taste
4 garlic cloves, peeled and minced
¼ cup heavy cream
3 cups ham, chopped
16 ounces cauliflower florets

Directions:
1.In a slow cooker, mix ham with stock, cheese, cauliflower, garlic powder, onion powder, salt, pepper, garlic, and heavy cream, stir, cover, and cook on high for 4 hours.
2.Stir, divide into bowls, and serve.

Nutrition: Calories: 306, Fat: 20.4, Fiber: 2.8, Carbohydrates: 8.4, Protein: 22.6

Veal Stew

Prep Time: 10 minutes **Cook Time:** 2 hours and 10 minutes
Servings: 12

Ingredients:
2 tablespoons avocado oil
3 pounds veal, cubed
1 onion, peeled and chopped
1 garlic clove, peeled and minced
Salt and ground black pepper, to taste
1 cup water
1½ cups marsala wine
10 ounces canned tomato paste
4 oz butternut squash peeled, and chopped
7 ounces mushrooms, chopped
3 egg yolks
½ cup heavy cream
2 teaspoons dried oregano

Directions:
1.Heat a pot with oil over medium–high heat, add veal, stir, and brown it for a few minutes.
2.Add garlic and onion, stir, and cook for 2–3 minutes.
3.Add wine, water, oregano, tomato paste, mushrooms, squash, salt, and pepper, stir, bring to a boil, cover, reduce the heat to low, and cook for 1 hour and 45 minutes.
4.In a bowl, mix cream with egg yolks, and whisk.
5.Pour into pot, stir, cook for 15 minutes, add more salt and pepper if needed, divide into bowls, and serve.

Nutrition: Calories: 284, Fat: 9.6, Fiber: 1.7, Carbohydrates: 8.9, Protein: 24.3

Veal with Tomatoes

Prep Time: 10 minutes **Cook Time:** 40 minutes
Servings: 4

Ingredients:
4 medium veal leg steaks
A drizzle of avocado oil
2 garlic cloves, peeled and minced
1 onion, peeled and chopped
Salt and ground black pepper, to taste
2 teaspoons fresh sage, chopped
15 ounces canned diced tomatoes
2 tablespoons fresh parsley, chopped
1 ounce semi–soft cheese, sliced
Green beans, steamed, for serving

Directions:
1.Heat a pan with oil over medium–high heat, add veal, cook for 2 minutes on each side, and transfer to a baking dish.
2.Return pan to heat, add onion, stir, and cook for 4 minutes.
3.Add sage and garlic, stir, and cook for 1 minute. Add tomatoes, stir, bring to a boil, and cook for 10 minutes.
4.Pour over the veal; add cheese and parsley, place in an oven at 350°F and bake for 20 minutes.
5.Divide on plates and serve.

Nutrition: Calories: 759, Fat: 54.1, Fiber: 17.1, Carbohydrates: 37.6, Protein: 44

Veal Parmesan

Prep Time: 10 minutes **Cook Time:** 1 hour and 10 minutes **Servings:** 6

Ingredients:
8 veal cutlets
⅔ cup Parmesan cheese, grated
8 provolone cheese slices
Salt and ground black pepper, to taste
5 cups tomato sauce
A pinch of garlic salt
Vegetable oil cooking spray
2 tablespoons butter
2 tablespoons coconut oil, melted
1 teaspoon Italian seasoning

Directions:
1.Season veal cutlets with salt, pepper, and garlic salt.
2.Heat a pan with butter and oil over medium–high heat, add veal, and cook until brown on all sides.
3.Line a baking dish with cooking spray and spread half of the tomato sauce on the bottom of the dish.
4.Add veal cutlets, then sprinkle with Italian seasoning and spread rest of the sauce.
5.Cover dish, place in an oven at 350°F and bake for 40 minutes.
6.Uncover dish, spread with provolone cheese, sprinkle with Parmesan cheese, place in an oven again and bake for 15 minutes.
7.Divide on plates and serve.

Nutrition: Calories: 620, Fat: 37.6, Fiber: 3.1, Carbohydrates: 12.3, Protein: 58.7

Veal Piccata

Prep Time: 10 minutes **Cook Time:** 15 minutes
Servings: 2

Ingredients:
2 tablespoons butter
¼ cup white wine
¼ cup chicken stock
1½ tablespoons capers
1 garlic clove, peeled and minced
8 ounces veal scallops
Salt and ground black pepper, to taste

Directions:
1.Heat a pan with half of the butter over medium–high heat, add veal cutlets, season with salt and pepper, cook for 1 minute on each side, and transfer to a plate.
2.Heat the pan again over medium heat, add garlic, stir, and cook for 1 minute.
3.Add wine, stir, and simmer for 2 minutes.
4.Add stock, capers, salt, pepper, remaining butter, and return the veal to pan.
5.Stir everything, cover the pan, and cook piccata on medium–low heat until veal is tender.

Nutrition: Calories: 434, Fat: 14.4, Fiber: 0.8, Carbohydrates: 10.6, Protein: 57.9

Baked Sausage and Kale

Prep Time: 5 minutes **Cook Time:** 30 minutes
Servings: 4

Ingredients:
1 cup onion, peeled and chopped
1½ pound Italian pork sausage, sliced
½ cup red bell pepper, seeded and chopped
Salt and ground black pepper, to taste
5 pounds kale, chopped
1 teaspoon garlic, minced
¼ cup red chili pepper, chopped
1 cup water

Directions:
1.Heat a pan over medium–high heat, add sausage, stir, reduce heat to medium, and cook for 10 minutes.
2.Add onions, stir, and cook for 3–4 minutes. Add bell pepper and garlic, stir, and cook for 1 minute.
3.Add kale, chili pepper, salt, pepper, and water, stir, and cook for 10 minutes.
4.Divide on plates and serve.

Nutrition: Calories: 872, Fat: 48.3, Fiber: 9.3, Carbohydrates: 63.1, Protein: 50.4

Sausage with Tomato and Cheese

Prep Time: 10 minutes **Cook Time:** 30 minutes
Servings: 4

Ingredients:
2 ounces coconut oil, melted
2 pounds sugar-free pork sausage, chopped
1 onion, peeled and sliced
4 sundried tomatoes, sliced thin
Salt and ground black pepper, to taste
½ pound gouda cheese, grated
3 yellow bell peppers, seeded and chopped
3 orange bell peppers, seeded and chopped
A pinch of red pepper flakes
½ cup parsley, sliced thin

Directions:
1.Heat a pan with oil over medium–high heat, add sausage slices, stir, cook for 3 minutes on each side, transfer to a plate, and set aside.
2.Heat the pan again over medium heat, add onion, bell peppers, and tomatoes, stir, and cook for 5 minutes.
3.Add pepper flakes, salt, and pepper, stir well, cook for 1 minute, and take off heat.
4.Arrange the sausage slices into a baking dish, add bell peppers mixture on top, add parsley and Gouda cheese, place in an oven at 350°F and bake for 15 minutes.
5.Divide on plates and serve hot.

Nutrition: Calories: 1176, Fat: 94.7, Fiber: 3.7, Carbohydrates: 7.7, Protein: 61.2

Sausage Salad

Prep Time: 10 minutes **Cook Time:** 7 minutes
Servings: 4

Ingredients:
8 pork sausage links, sliced
1 pound mixed cherry tomatoes, cut in half
4 cups baby spinach
1 tablespoon avocado oil
1 pound mozzarella cheese, cubed
2 tablespoons lemon juice
⅔ cup basil pesto
Salt and ground black pepper, to taste

Directions:
1.Heat a pan with the over medium–high heat, add sausage slices, stir, and cook them for 4 minutes on each side.
2.In a salad bowl, mix spinach with mozzarella cheese, tomatoes, salt, pepper, lemon juice, and pesto, and toss to coat.
3.Add sausage pieces, toss again, and serve.

Nutrition: Calories: 150, Fat: 9.7, Fiber: 2.9, Carbohydrates: 7.8, Protein: 10.1

Roasted Pork Sausage

Prep Time: 10 minutes **Cook Time:** 1 hour
Servings: 6

Ingredients:
3 red bell peppers, seeded and chopped
2 pounds Italian pork sausage, sliced
Salt and ground black pepper, to taste
2 pounds Portobello mushrooms, sliced
2 sweet onions, peeled and chopped
1 tablespoon swerve
A drizzle of olive oil

Directions:
1.In a baking dish, mix sausage slices with oil, salt, pepper, bell pepper, mushrooms, onion, and swerve.
2.Toss to coat, place in oven at 300ºF and bake for 1 hour. Divide on plates and serve hot.

Nutrition: Calories: 585, Fat: 43.1, Fiber: 1.6, Carbohydrates: 11.8, Protein: 34.2

Sausage and Pepper Soup

Prep Time: 10 minutes **Cook Time:** 1 hour and 10 minutes
Servings: 6

Ingredients:
1 tablespoon avocado oil
32 ounces pork sausage meat
10 ounces canned tomatoes, and jalapeños, chopped
10 ounces spinach
1 green bell pepper, seeded and chopped
4 cups beef stock
1 teaspoon onion powder
Salt and ground black pepper, to taste
1 tablespoon cumin
1 tablespoon chili powder
1 teaspoon garlic powder
1 teaspoon Italian seasoning

Directions:
1.Heat a pot with oil over medium heat, add sausage, stir, and brown for a couple of minutes on all sides.
2.Add green bell pepper, salt, and pepper, stir, and cook for 3 minutes. Add tomatoes and jalapeños, stir, and cook for 2 minutes. Add spinach, stir, cover, and cook for 7 minutes.
3.Add stock, onion powder, garlic powder, chili powder, cumin, salt, pepper, and Italian seasoning, stir, cover the pot, and cook for 30 minutes.
4.Uncover pot and cook soup for 15 minutes. Divide into bowls and serve.

Nutrition: Calories: 538, Fat: 46.5, Fiber: 2, Carbohydrates: 5.3, Protein: 21.2

Italian Sausage Soup

Prep Time: 10 minutes **Cook Time:** 30 minutes
Servings: 12

Ingredients:
½ gallon chicken stock
A drizzle of avocado oil
1 cup heavy cream
10 ounces spinach
6 bacon slices, chopped
1 pound radishes, chopped
2 garlic cloves, peeled and minced
Salt and ground black pepper, to taste
A pinch of red pepper flakes
1 onion, peeled and chopped
1½ pounds hot pork sausage, chopped

Directions:
1.Heat a pot with a drizzle of avocado oil over medium–high heat, add sausage, onion, and garlic, stir, and brown for a few minutes.
2.Add stock, spinach, radishes, stir, and bring to a simmer.
3.Add bacon, cream, salt, pepper, red pepper flakes, stir, and cook for 20 minutes. Divide into bowls and serve.

Nutrition: Calories: 586, Fat: 43.9, Fiber: 1.3, Carbohydrates: 9.3, Protein: 37

Vegetable

Avocado Salad

Prep Time: 10 minutes **Cook Time:** 0 minutes
Servings: 4

Ingredients:
2 avocados, pitted, and mashed
Salt and ground black pepper, to taste
¼ teaspoon lemon stevia
1 tablespoon white vinegar
Juice from 2 limes
¼ cup onion, chopped
¼ cup fresh cilantro, chopped
2 tablespoons olive oil
For coleslaw mix
1/4 small red cabbage
1/2 small green cabbage
1/2 carrot, shredded
zest of 1/2 lemon
1/4 cup lemon juice
1/4 cup olive oil
1 tablespoon stevia
1 teaspoon salt.

Directions:
1.Make coleslaw mixture in a salad bowl.
2.Add avocado mash and onions and toss to coat.
3.In a bowl, mix lime juice with salt, pepper, oil, vinegar, stevia, and stir well.
4.Add this to salad, toss to coat, sprinkle cilantro, and serve.

Nutrition: Calories: 481, Fat: 45.2, Fiber: 12.2, Carbohydrates: 22.6, Protein: 4.6

Avocado and Egg Salad

Prep Time: 10 minutes **Cook Time:** 7 minutes
Servings: 4

Ingredients:
4 cups mixed lettuce leaves, torn
4 eggs
1 avocado, pitted, and sliced
¼ cup mayonnaise
2 teaspoons mustard
2 garlic cloves, peeled and minced
1 tablespoon fresh chives, chopped
Salt and ground black pepper, to taste

Directions:
1.Put water in a saucepan, add some salt, eggs, bring to a boil over medium–high heat, boil for 7 minutes, drain, cool, peel, and chop them.
2.In a salad bowl, mix lettuce eggs and avocado.
3.Add chives and garlic, some salt, and pepper, and toss to coat.
4.In a bowl, mix mustard with mayonnaise, salt, pepper, and stir well. Add this to the salad, toss well, and serve.

Nutrition: Calories: 278, Fat: 19.6, Fiber: 6.7, Carbohydrates: 15.3, Protein: 10.2

Avocado and Cucumber Salad

Prep Time: 10 minutes **Cook Time:** 0 minutes
Servings: 4

Ingredients:
1 onion, peeled and sliced
1 cucumber, sliced
2 avocados, pitted, peeled, and chopped
1 pound cherry tomatoes, halved
2 tablespoons olive oil
¼ cup fresh cilantro, chopped
2 tablespoons lemon juice
Salt and ground black pepper, to taste

Directions:
1.In a large salad bowl, mix tomatoes with cucumber, onion, avocado, and stir.
2.Add oil, salt, pepper, lemon juice, and toss to coat well. Serve cold with cilantro on top.

Nutrition: Calories: 310, Fat: 27, Fiber: 9.1, Carbohydrates: 18.6, Protein: 3.8

Arugula Soup

Prep Time: 10 minutes **Cook Time:** 13 minutes
Servings: 6

Ingredients:
1 onion, peeled and chopped
1 tablespoon olive oil
2 garlic cloves, peeled and minced
½ cup coconut milk
10 ounces baby arugula
2 tablespoons fresh mint, chopped, and
2 tablespoons fresh tarragon, chopped
2 tablespoons fresh parsley, chopped
2 tablespoons fresh chives, chopped
4 tablespoons coconut milk yogurt
6 cups chicken stock
Salt and ground black pepper, to taste

Directions:
1.Heat a saucepan with oil over medium–high heat, add onion and garlic, stir, and cook for 5 minutes.
2.Add stock, milk, stir, and bring to a simmer.
3.Add arugula, tarragon, parsley, mint, stir, and cook for 6 minutes.
4.Add coconut yogurt, salt, pepper, chives, stir, cook for 2 minutes, divide into soup bowls, and serve.

Nutrition: Calories: 186, Fat: 11.4, Fiber: 7.9, Carbohydrates: 20.9, Protein: 4.2

Avocado and Bacon Soup

Prep Time: 10 minutes **Cook Time:** 10 minutes
Servings: 4

Ingredients:
2 avocados, pitted, and cut in half
4 cups chicken stock
⅓ cup fresh cilantro, chopped
Juice of ½ lime
1 teaspoon garlic powder
½ pound bacon, cooked, and chopped
Salt and ground black pepper, to taste

Directions:
1.Put the stock in a saucepan and bring to a boil over medium–high heat.
2.In a blender, mix avocados with garlic powder, cilantro, lime juice, salt, pepper, and blend well. Add to the stock and blend using an immersion blender.
3.Add bacon, more salt and pepper, stir, cook for 3 minutes, ladle into soup bowls, and serve.

Nutrition: Calories: 524, Fat: 43.9, Fiber: 6.8, Carbohydrates: 10.7, Protein: 23.7

Arugula and Broccoli Soup

Prep Time: 10 minutes **Cook Time:** 20 minutes
Servings: 4

Ingredients:
1 onion, peeled and chopped
1 tablespoon olive oil
1 garlic clove, peeled and minced
1 broccoli head, separated into florets
Salt and ground black pepper, to taste
2, and ½ cups vegetable stock
1 teaspoon cumin
Juice of ½ lemon
1 cup arugula leaves

Directions:
1.Heat a saucepan with the over medium–high heat, add onions, stir, and cook for 4 minutes.
2.Add garlic, stir, and cook for 1 minute.
3.Add broccoli, cumin, salt, and pepper, stir, and cook for 4 minutes. Add stock, stir, and cook for 8 minutes.
4.Blend soup using an immersion blender, add half of arugula, and blend again.
5.Add rest of the arugula, stir, and heat up soup again.
6.Add lemon juice, stir, ladle into soup bowls, and serve.

Nutrition: Calories: 74, Fat: 4.9, Fiber: 2.5, Carbohydrates: 8.8, Protein: 2.5

Avocado Soup

Prep Time: 10 minutes **Cook Time:** 10 minutes
Servings: 4

Ingredients:
2 avocados, pitted, peeled, and chopped
3 cups chicken stock
2 scallions, chopped
Salt and ground black pepper, to taste
2 tablespoons butter
⅔ cup heavy cream

Directions:
1.Heat a saucepan with butter over medium heat, add scallions, stir, and cook for 2 minutes.
2.Add 2½ cups stock, stir, and simmer for 3 minutes.
3.In a blender, mix avocados with rest of the stock, salt, pepper, heavy cream, and pulse well. Add to the pan, stir well, cook for 2 minutes, and season with more salt and pepper.
4.Stir, ladle into soup bowls, and serve.

Nutrition: Calories: 335, Fat: 33.2, Fiber: 6.9, Carbohydrates: 10.3, Protein: 3

Thai Avocado Soup

Prep Time: 10 minutes **Cook Time:** 10 minutes
Servings: 4

Ingredients:
1 cup coconut milk
2 teaspoons Thai green curry paste
1 avocado, pitted, peeled, and chopped
1 tablespoon fresh cilantro, chopped
Salt and ground black pepper, to taste
2 cups vegetable stock
Lime wedges, for serving

Directions:
1.In a blender, mix avocado with salt, pepper, curry paste, coconut milk, and pulse well.
2.Transfer to a saucepan and heat over medium heat.
3.Add stock, stir, bring to a simmer, and cook for 5 minutes.
4.Add cilantro, more salt and pepper, stir, cook for 1 minute, ladle into soup bowls, and serve with lime wedges.

Nutrition: Calories: 250, Fat: 24.9, Fiber: 5, Carbohydrates: 8.2, Protein: 2.4

Broccoli Stew

Prep Time: 10 minutes **Cook Time:** 40 minutes
Servings: 4

Ingredients:
1 broccoli head, separated into florets
2 teaspoons coriander seeds
A drizzle of olive oil
1 onion, peeled and chopped
Salt and ground black pepper, to taste
A pinch of red pepper, crushed
1 small ginger piece, peeled, and chopped
1 garlic clove, peeled and minced
28 ounces canned sugar-free pureed tomatoes

Directions:
1.Put water in a saucepan, add salt, bring to a boil over medium–high heat, add broccoli florets, steam for 2 minutes, transfer to a bowl filled with ice water, drain them, and leave aside.
2.Heat a pan over medium–high heat, add coriander seeds, toast them for 4 minutes, transfer to a grinder, grind, and set aside as well.
3.Heat a pot with oil over medium heat, add onions, salt, pepper, red pepper, stir, and cook for 7 minutes.
4.Add ginger, garlic, and coriander seeds, stir, and cook for 3 minutes.
5.Add tomatoes, bring to a boil, and simmer for 10 minutes.
6.Add broccoli, stir and cook stew for 12 minutes. Divide into bowls and serve.

Nutrition: Calories: 152, Fat: 0.9, Fiber: 8.8, Carbohydrates: 4.1, Protein: 7.9

Arugula Salad

Prep Time: 10 minutes **Cook Time:** 0 minutes
Servings: 4

Ingredients:
1 white onion, peeled and chopped
1 tablespoon vinegar
1 cup hot water
1 bunch baby arugula
¼ cup walnuts, chopped
2 tablespoons fresh cilantro, chopped
2 garlic cloves, peeled and minced
2 tablespoons olive oil
Salt and ground black pepper, to taste
1 tablespoon lemon juice

Directions:
1.In a bowl, mix water with vinegar, add onion, set aside for 5 minutes, and drain.
2.In a salad bowl, mix arugula with walnuts and onion, and stir.
3.Add garlic, salt, pepper, lemon juice, cilantro, and oil, toss well, and serve.

Nutrition: Calories: 123, Fat: 11.7, Fiber: 1.2, Carbohydrates: 4, Protein: 2.4

Zucchini Cream

Prep Time: 10 minutes **Cook Time:** 25 minutes
Servings: 8

Ingredients:
6 zucchini, cut in half and sliced
Salt and ground black pepper, to taste
1 tablespoon butter
28 ounces vegetable stock
1 teaspoon dried oregano
½ cup onion, chopped
3 garlic cloves, peeled and minced
2 ounces Parmesan cheese, grated
¾ cup heavy cream

Directions:
1.Heat a saucepan with the butter over medium–high heat, add onion, stir, and cook for 4 minutes.
2.Add garlic, stir, and cook for 2 minutes.
3.Add zucchini, stir, and cook for 3 minutes.
4.Add stock, stir, bring to a boil, and simmer over medium heat for 15 minutes.
5.Add oregano, salt, pepper, stir, take off heat, and blend using an immersion blender.
6.Heat soup again, add heavy cream, stir, and bring to a simmer.
7.Add Parmesan cheese, stir, take off heat, ladle into bowls, and serve.

Nutrition: Calories: 109, Fat: 7.5, Fiber: 2.4, Carbohydrates: 7.5, Protein: 4.9

Puréed Broccoli and Cauliflower

Prep Time: 10 minutes **Cook Time:** 15 minutes
Servings: 5

Ingredients:
1 cauliflower head, separated into florets
1 broccoli head, separated into florets
Salt and ground black pepper, to taste
2 garlic cloves, peeled and minced
2 bacon slices, chopped
2 tablespoons butter

Directions:
1.Heat a saucepan with butter over medium–high heat, add garlic and bacon, stir, and cook for 3 minutes.
2.Add cauliflower and broccoli florets, stir, and cook for 2 minutes.
3.Add water to cover them, cover pot, and simmer for 10 minutes.
4.Add salt and pepper, stir again, and blend soup using an immersion blender.
5.Simmer for a couple minutes over medium heat, ladle into bowls, and serve.

Nutrition: Calories: 128, Fat: 8.2, Fiber: 3.7, Carbohydrates: 9.4, Protein: 6.6

Watercress Soup

Prep Time: 10 minutes **Cook Time:** 10 minutes **Servings:** 4

Ingredients:
6 cup chicken stock
¼ cup sherry
2 teaspoons coconut aminos
6, and ½ cups watercress
Salt and ground black pepper, to taste
2 teaspoons sesame seed
3 shallots, peeled and chopped
3 egg whites, whisked

Directions:
1.Put the stock into a pot, mix with salt, pepper, sherry, and coconut aminos, stir, and bring to a boil over medium–high heat.
2.Add shallots, watercress, egg whites, stir, bring to a boil, divide into bowls, and serve with sesame seeds sprinkled on top.

Nutrition: Calories: 73, Fat: 1.7, Fiber: 0.2, Carbohydrates: 6.7, Protein: 5.9

Bok Choy Soup

Prep Time: 10 minutes **Cook Time:** 15 minutes **Servings:** 4

Ingredients:
3 cups beef stock
1 onion, peeled and chopped
1 bunch bok choy, chopped
1½ cups mushrooms, chopped
Salt and ground black pepper, to taste
½ tablespoon red pepper flakes
3 tablespoons coconut aminos
3 tablespoons Parmesan cheese, grated
2 tablespoons Worcestershire sauce
2 bacon strips, chopped

Directions:
1.Heat a saucepan over medium–high heat, add bacon, stir, cook until crispy, transfer to paper towels and drain the grease.
2.Heat the saucepan again over medium heat, add mushrooms and onions, stir, and cook for 5 minutes.
3.Add stock, bok choy, coconut aminos, salt, pepper, pepper flakes, and Worcestershire sauce, stir, cover, and cook until bok choy is tender.
4.Ladle the soup into bowls, sprinkle Parmesan cheese, and bacon, and serve.

Nutrition: Calories: 100, Fat: 3.5, Fiber: 1.9, Carbohydrates: 8.1, Protein: 8.5

Collard Greens and Ham

Prep Time: 10 minutes **Cook Time:** 1 hour and 40 minutes **Servings:** 4

Ingredients:
4 ounces ham, boneless, cooked, and chopped
1 tablespoon olive oil
2 pounds collard greens, cut in medium strips
1 teaspoon red pepper flakes
Salt and ground black pepper, to taste
2 cups chicken stock
1 onion, peeled and chopped
4 ounces dry white wine
1 ounce salt pork
¼ cup apple cider vinegar
½ cup butter, melted

Directions:
1.Heat a pan with oil over medium–high heat, add ham and onion, stir, and cook for 4 minutes.
2.Add salt pork, collard greens, stock, vinegar, wine, stir, and bring to a boil.
3.Reduce heat, cover pan, and cook for 1 hour and 30 minutes, stirring from occasionally.
4.Add butter, discard the salt pork, stir, cook everything for 10 minutes, divide on plates, and serve.

Nutrition: Calories: 430, Fat: 35.6, Fiber: 8.4, Carbohydrates: 17.4, Protein: 11.2

Bok Choy Stir-fry

Prep Time: 10 minutes **Cook Time:** 7 minutes
Servings: 2

Ingredients:
2 garlic cloves, peeled and minced
2 cup bok choy, chopped
2 bacon slices, chopped
Salt and ground black pepper, to taste
A drizzle of avocado oil

Directions:
1.Heat a pan with oil over medium heat, add bacon, stir, and brown until crispy, transfer to paper towels, and drain the grease.
2.Return the pan to medium heat, add garlic and bok choy, stir, and cook for 4 minutes.
3.Add salt, pepper, and return the bacon to pan, stir, cook for 1 minute, divide on plates, and serve.

Nutrition: Calories: 116, Fat: 8.1, Fiber: 0.8, Carbohydrates: 2.8, Protein: 8.3

Cream of Celery Soup

Prep Time: 10 minutes **Cook Time:** 40 minutes
Servings: 4

Ingredients:
1 bunch celery, chopped
Salt and ground black pepper, to taste
3 bay leaves
½ garlic head, peeled, and chopped
2 onions, peeled and chopped
4 cups chicken stock
¾ cup heavy cream
2 tablespoons butter

Directions:
1.Heat a saucepan with butter over medium–high heat, add onions, salt, and pepper, stir, and cook for 5 minutes.
2.Add bay leaves, garlic, and celery, stir, and cook for 15 minutes.
3.Add stock, more salt and pepper, stir, cover pan, reduce the heat, and simmer for 20 minutes.
4.Add cream, stir, and blend everything using an immersion blender. Ladle into soup bowls and serve.

Nutrition: Calories: 191, Fat: 15, Fiber: 2.8, Carbohydrates: 12.9, Protein: 3.1

Collard Greens and Poached Eggs

Prep Time: 10 minutes **Cook Time:** 15 minutes
Servings: 6

Ingredients:
1 tablespoon chipotle, mashed
6 eggs
3 tablespoons butter
1 onion, peeled and chopped
2 garlic cloves, peeled and minced
6 bacon slices, chopped
3 bunches collard greens, chopped
½ cup chicken stock
Salt and ground black pepper, to taste
1 tablespoon lime juice
Cheddar cheese, grated, for serving

Directions:
1.Heat a pan over medium–high heat, add bacon, cook until crispy, transfer to paper towels, drain grease, and leave aside.
2.Heat the pan again over medium heat, add garlic and onion, stir, and cook for 2 minutes.
3.Return bacon to the pan, stir, and cook for 3 minutes.
4.Add chipotle, collard greens, salt, and pepper, stir, and cook for 10 minutes.
5.Add stock and lime juice, and stir.
6.Make 6 holes in collard greens mixture, divide butter, crack an egg in each hole, cover the pan, and cook until eggs are done.
7.Divide this on plates and serve with cheddar cheese sprinkled on top.

Nutrition: Calories: 235, Fat: 18.4, Fiber: 1.4, Carbohydrates: 4.4, Protein: 13.6

Celery Soup

Prep Time: 10 minutes **Cook Time:** 25 minutes
Servings: 8

Ingredients:
26 ounces celery leaves, and stalks, chopped
1 tablespoon dried onion flakes
Salt and ground black pepper, to taste
3 teaspoons fenugreek powder
3 teaspoons vegetable stock powder
10 ounces sour cream

Directions:
1.Put the celery into a saucepan, add the water to cover, add onion flakes, salt, pepper, stock powder, and fenugreek powder, stir, bring to a boil over medium heat, and simmer for 20 minutes.
2.Use an immersion blender to make the cream, add sour cream, more salt and pepper, and blend again.
3.Heat up soup again over medium heat, ladle into bowls, and serve.

Nutrition: Calories: 99, Fat: 7.9, Fiber: 1.9, Carbohydrates: 5.8, Protein: 2.1

Celery Stew

Prep Time: 10 minutes **Cook Time:** 30 minutes
Servings: 6

Ingredients:
1 celery bunch, chopped
1 onion, peeled and chopped
1 bunch green onion, peeled and chopped
4 garlic cloves, peeled and minced
Salt and ground black pepper, to taste
1 fresh parsley bunch, chopped
2 fresh mint bunches, chopped
3 dried Persian lemons, pricked with a fork
2 cups water
2 teaspoons chicken bouillon
4 tablespoons olive oil

Directions:
1.Heat a saucepan with oil over medium–high heat, add onion, green onions, and garlic, stir, and cook for 6 minutes.
2.Add celery, Persian lemons, chicken bouillon, salt, pepper, water, stir, cover pan, and simmer on medium heat for 20 minutes.
3.Add parsley and mint, stir, and cook for 10 minutes. Divide into bowls and serve.

Nutrition: Calories: 100, Fat: 9.5, Fiber: 1.4, Carbohydrates: 4.4, Protein: 0.9

Spinach Soup

Prep Time: 10 minutes **Cook Time:** 15 minutes
Servings: 8

Ingredients:
2 tablespoons butter
20 ounces spinach, chopped
1 teaspoon garlic, minced
Salt and ground black pepper, to taste
45 ounces chicken stock
½ teaspoon ground nutmeg
2 cups heavy cream
1 onion, peeled and chopped

Directions:
1.Heat a saucepan with butter over medium heat, add onion, stir, and cook for 4 minutes.
2.Add garlic, stir, and cook for 1 minute.
3.Add spinach and stock, stir, and cook for 5 minutes.
4.Blend soup with an immersion blender, and heat up the soup again.
5.Add salt, pepper, nutmeg, cream, stir, and cook for 5 minutes.
6.Ladle into bowls and serve.

Nutrition: Calories: 158, Fat: 14.7, Fiber: 1.9, Carbohydrates: 5.4, Protein: 3.3

Sautéed Mustard Greens

Prep Time: 10 minutes **Cook Time:** 20 minutes
Servings: 4

Ingredients:
2 garlic cloves, peeled and minced
1 tablespoon olive oil
2½ pounds collard greens, chopped
1 teaspoon lemon juice
1 tablespoon butter
Salt and ground black pepper, to taste

Directions:
1.Put some water in a saucepan, add salt, and bring to a simmer over medium heat.
2.Add greens, cover, and cook for 15 minutes.
3.Drain collard greens, press the liquid out, and put them in a bowl.
4.Heat a pan with oil and butter over medium–high heat, add collard greens, salt, pepper, and garlic.
5.Stir well and cook for 5 minutes.
6.Add more salt and pepper if needed, drizzle with lemon juice, stir, divide on plates, and serve.

Nutrition: Calories: 385, Fat: 14.7, Fiber: 39.3, Carbohydrates: 66, Protein: 26.3

Collard Greens and Tomatoes

Prep Time: 10 minutes **Cook Time:** 12 minutes
Servings: 5

Ingredients:
1 pound collard greens
3 bacon strips, chopped
¼ cup cherry tomatoes, halved
1 tablespoon apple cider vinegar
2 tablespoons chicken stock
Salt and ground black pepper, to taste

Directions:
1.Heat a pan over medium heat, add bacon, stir, and cook until it browns.
2.Add tomatoes, collard greens, vinegar, stock, salt, and pepper, stir, and cook for 8 minutes.
3.Add more salt, and pepper, stir again gently, divide on plates, and serve.

Nutrition: Calories: 63, Fat: 3.4, Fiber: 3.7, Carbohydrates: 6.6, Protein: 3.3

Mustard Greens and Spinach Soup

Prep Time: 10 minutes **Cook Time:** 15 minutes
Servings: 6

Ingredients:
½ teaspoon fenugreek seeds
1 teaspoon cumin seeds
1 tablespoon avocado oil
1 teaspoon coriander seeds
1 cup onion, chopped
1 tablespoon garlic, minced
1 tablespoon fresh ginger, grated
½ teaspoon turmeric
5 cups mustard greens, chopped
3 cups coconut milk
1 tablespoon jalapeño, chopped
5 cups spinach, torn
Salt and ground black pepper, to taste
2 teaspoons butter
½ teaspoon paprika

Directions:
1.Heat a saucepan with oil over medium–high heat, add coriander, fenugreek, cumin seeds, stir, and brown them for 2 minutes.
2.Add onions, stir, and cook for 3 minutes.
3.Add half of the garlic, jalapeños, ginger, turmeric, stir, and cook for 3 minutes.
4.Add mustard greens, spinach, stir, and sauté everything for 10 minutes.
5.Add milk, salt, and pepper, and blend the soup using an immersion blender.
6.Heat a pan with the butter over medium heat, add garlic, and paprika, stir well, and take off heat.
7.Heat the soup over medium heat, ladle into soup bowls, drizzle with butter and sprinkle with paprika, and serve.

Nutrition: Calories: 324, Fat: 30.6, Fiber: 5.6, Carbohydrates: 13.4, Protein: 5.3

Sautéed Mustard Greens

Prep Time: 5 minutes **Cook Time:** 15 minutes
Servings: 4

Ingredients:
2 garlic cloves, peeled and minced
1 pound mustard greens, torn
1 tablespoon olive oil
½ cup onion, sliced
Salt and ground black pepper, to taste
3 tablespoons vegetable stock
¼ teaspoon dark sesame oil

Directions:
1.Heat a pan with oil over medium heat, add onions, stir, and brown them for 10 minutes.
2.Add garlic, stir, and cook for 1 minute. Add stock, greens, salt, and pepper, stir, and cook for 5 minutes.
3.Add more salt and pepper, and sesame oil, toss to coat, divide on plates, and serve.

Nutrition: Calories: 70, Fat: 4, Fiber: 4.1, Carbohydrates: 7.5, Protein: 3.3

Collard Greens Soup

Prep Time: 10 minutes **Cook Time:** 40 minutes
Servings: 12

Ingredients:
1 teaspoon chili powder
1 tablespoon avocado oil
2 teaspoons smoked paprika
1 teaspoon cumin
1 onion, peeled and chopped
A pinch of red pepper flakes
10 cups water
3 celery stalks, chopped
10 oz butternut squash, peeled and chopped
15 ounces sugar-free canned diced tomatoes
2 tablespoons tamari sauce
6 ounces sagar-free tomato passata
2 tablespoons lemon juice
Salt and ground black pepper, to taste
6 cups collard greens, stems discarded
1 tablespoon swerve
1 teaspoon dried garlic
1 tablespoon herb seasoning

Directions:
1.Heat a pot with over medium–high heat, add cumin, pepper flakes, paprika, chili powder, and stir well.
2.Add celery, onion, squash, stir, and cook for 10 minutes.
3.Add tamari sauce, tomatoes, tomato passata, water, lemon juice, salt, pepper, herb seasoning, swerve, garlic granules, collard greens, stir, bring to a boil, cover, and cook for 30 minutes.
4.Stir again, ladle into bowls, and serve.

Nutrition: Calories: 384, Fat: 6.8, Fiber: 2.2, Carbohydrates: 7.1, Protein:16.6

Spring Greens Soup

Prep Time: 10 minutes **Cook Time:** 30 minutes
Servings: 4

Ingredients:
2 cups mustard greens, chopped
2 cups collard greens, chopped
3 quarts vegetable stock
1 onion, peeled and chopped
Salt and ground black pepper, to taste
2 tablespoons coconut aminos
2 teaspoons fresh ginger, grated

Directions:
1.Put the stock into a saucepan and bring to a simmer over medium–high heat.
2.Add mustard, collard greens, onion, salt, pepper, coconut aminos, ginger, stir, cover the pan, and cook for 30 minutes.
3.Blend the soup using an immersion blender, add more salt, and pepper, heat up over medium heat, ladle into soup bowls, and serve.

Nutrition: Calories: 35, Fat: 0.4, Fiber: 2.8, Carbohydrates: 7, Protein: 1.9

Roasted Asparagus

Prep Time: 10 minutes **Cook Time:** 10 minutes
Servings: 3

Ingredients:
1 asparagus bunch, trimmed
3 teaspoons avocado oil
A splash of lemon juice
Salt and ground black pepper, to taste
1 tablespoon fresh oregano, chopped

Directions:
1.Spread asparagus spears on a lined baking sheet, season with salt, pepper, drizzle with oil and lemon juice, sprinkle with oregano, and toss to coat well.
2.Place in an oven at 425ºF and bake for 10 minutes. Divide on plates and serve.

Nutrition: Calories: 14, Fat: 0.6, Fiber: 1, Carbohydrates: 1.8, Protein: 0.9

Asparagus Fries

Prep Time: 10 minutes **Cook Time:** 10 minutes
Servings: 2

Ingredients:
¼ cup Parmesan cheese, grated
16 asparagus spears, trimmed
1 egg, whisked
½ teaspoon onion powder
2 ounces pork rinds

Directions:
1.Crush pork rinds and put them in a bowl.
2.Add onion powder and cheese and stir.
3.Roll asparagus spears in egg, then dip them in pork rind mixture, and arrange them all on a lined baking sheet.
4.Place in oven at 425ºF and bake for 10 minutes.
5.Divide on plates and serve them with sour cream on the side.

Nutrition: Calories: 279, Fat: 15.6, Fiber: 4.1, Carbohydrates: 8.6, Protein: 29.8

Asparagus Frittata

Prep Time: 10 minutes **Cook Time:** 15 minutes
Servings: 4

Ingredients:
¼ cup onion, chopped
A drizzle of olive oil
1 pound asparagus spears, cut into 1–inch pieces
Salt and ground black pepper, to taste
4 eggs, whisked
1 cup cheddar cheese, grated

Directions:
1.Heat a pan with oil over medium–high heat, add onions, stir, and cook for 3 minutes.
2.Add asparagus, stir, and cook for 6 minutes. Add eggs, stir, and cook for 3 minutes.
3.Add salt and pepper, sprinkle with cheese, place in oven, and broil for 3 minutes.
4.Divide frittata on plates and serve.

Nutrition: Calories: 202, Fat: 13.9, Fiber: 2.5, Carbohydrates: 5.8, Protein: 15.1

Alfalfa Sprouts Salad

Prep Time: 10 minutes **Cook Time:** 0 minutes
Servings: 4

Ingredients:
1½ teaspoons dark sesame oil
4 cups alfalfa sprouts
Salt and ground black pepper, to taste
1½ teaspoons grape seed oil
¼ cup coconut milk yogurt

Directions:
1.In a salad bowl, mix sprouts with salt, pepper, sesame oil, grape seed oil, coconut yogurt, toss to coat, divide on plates, and serve.

Nutrition: Calories: 83, Fat: 7.6, Fiber: 1.8, Carbohydrates: 3.4, Protein: 1.6

Creamy Asparagus

Prep Time: 10 minutes **Cook Time:** 15 minutes
Servings: 3

Ingredients:
10 ounces asparagus spears, cut into medium–sized pieces, and steamed
Salt and ground black pepper, to taste
2 tablespoons Parmesan cheese, grated
⅓ cup Monterey jack cheese, shredded
2 tablespoons mustard
2 ounces cream cheese
⅓ cup heavy cream
3 tablespoons bacon, cooked and crumbled

Directions:
1.Heat a pan with mustard, heavy cream, cream cheese over medium heat and stir well.
2.Add Monterey Jack cheese, Parmesan cheese, stir, and cook until it melts.
3.Add half of the bacon, and asparagus, stir, and cook for 3 minutes.
4.Add rest of the bacon, plus salt and pepper, stir, cook for 5 minutes, divide on plates, and serve.

Nutrition: Calories: 346, Fat: 27.5, Fiber: 3.1, Carbohydrates: 7.8, Protein:18.8

Asparagus and Browned Butter

Prep Time: 10 minutes **Cook Time:** 15 minutes
Servings: 4

Ingredients:
5 ounces butter
1 tablespoon avocado oil
1½ pounds asparagus, trimmed
1½ tablespoons lemon juice
A pinch of cayenne pepper
8 tablespoons sour cream
Salt and ground black pepper, to taste
3 ounces Parmesan cheese, grated
4 eggs

Directions:
1.Heat a pan with 2 ounces butter over medium–high heat, add eggs, some salt and pepper, stir, and scramble them.
2.Transfer eggs to a blender, add Parmesan cheese, sour cream, salt, pepper, cayenne pepper, and blend everything well.
3.Heat a pan with oil over medium–high heat, add asparagus, salt, pepper, roast for a few minutes, transfer to a plate, and set aside.
4.Heat the pan again with rest of butter over medium–high heat, stir until brown, take off heat, add lemon juice, and stir well.
5.Heat the butter again, return asparagus to pan, toss to coat, heat up, and divide on plates.
6.Add blended eggs on top and serve.

Nutrition: Calories: 566, Fat: 43.9, Fiber: 13.3, Carbohydrates: 26.5, Protein: 27.2

Creamy Radishes

Prep Time: 10 minutes **Cook Time:** 25 minutes
Servings: 1

Ingredients:
7 ounces radishes, cut in half
2 tablespoons sour cream
2 bacon slices
1 tablespoon green onion, peeled and chopped
1 tablespoon cheddar cheese, grated
Cayenne pepper powder, to taste
Salt and ground black pepper, to taste

Directions:
1.Put the radishes into a saucepan, add water to cover, bring to a boil over medium heat, cook them for 10 minutes and drain.
2.Heat a pan over medium–high heat, add bacon, cook until crispy, transfer to paper towels, drain the grease, crumble, and leave aside.
3.Return pan to medium heat, add radishes, stir, and sauté them for 7 minutes.
4.Add onion, salt, pepper, cayenne pepper powder, sour cream, stir, and cook for 7 minutes.
5.Transfer to a plate, top with crumbled bacon and cheddar cheese, and serve.

Nutrition: Calories: 319, Fat: 23.5, Fiber: 3.3, Carbohydrates: 8.8, Protein: 18.1

Roasted Radishes

Prep Time: 10 minutes **Cook Time:** 35 minutes
Servings: 2

Ingredients:
2 cups radishes, cut in quarters
Salt and ground black pepper, to taste
2 tablespoons butter, melted
1 tablespoon fresh chives, chopped
1 tablespoon lemon zest

Directions:
1.Spread radishes on a lined baking sheet.
2.Add salt, pepper, chives, lemon zest, butter, toss to coat, and bake in the oven at 375ºF for 35 minutes.
3.Divide on plates and serve.

Nutrition: Calories: 123, Fat: 11.7, Fiber: 2.1, Carbohydrates: 4.6, Protein: 1

Crispy Radishes

Prep Time: 10 minutes **Cook Time:** 20 minutes
Servings: 4

Ingredients:
Vegetable oil cooking spray
15 radishes, sliced
Salt and ground black pepper, to taste
1 tablespoon fresh chives, chopped

Directions:
1.Arrange radish slices on a lined baking sheet and spray with cooking oil.
2.Season with salt and pepper, sprinkle with chives, place in an oven at 375ºF, and bake for 10 minutes.
3.Flip them and bake for 10 minutes. Serve cold.

Nutrition: Calories: 63, Fat: 6.8, Fiber: 0.3, Carbohydrates: 0.6, Protein: 0.1

Radish Hash Browns

Prep Time: 10 minutes **Cook Time:** 10 minutes
Servings: 4

Ingredients:
½ teaspoon onion powder
1 pound radishes, shredded
½ teaspoon garlic powder
Salt and ground black pepper, to taste
4 eggs
⅓ cup Parmesan cheese, grated

Directions:
1.In a bowl, mix radishes with salt, pepper, onion, garlic powder, eggs, Parmesan cheese, and stir well.
2.Spread on a lined baking sheet, place in an oven at 375ºF and bake for 10 minutes.
3.Divide the hash browns on plates and serve.

Nutrition: Calories: 104, Fat: 6, Fiber: 1.8, Carbohydrates: 4.5, Protein: 8.6

Radish Soup

Prep Time: 10 minutes **Cook Time:** 20 minutes
Servings: 4

Ingredients:
2 bunches radishes, cut in quarters
Salt and ground black pepper, to taste
6 cups chicken stock
2 stalks celery, chopped
3 tablespoons coconut oil
6 garlic cloves, peeled and minced
1 onion, peeled and chopped

Directions:
1.Heat a saucepan with oil over medium heat, add onion, celery, garlic, stir, and cook for 5 minutes.
2.Add radishes, stock, salt, and pepper, stir, bring to a boil, cover, and simmer for 15 minutes.
3.Divide into soup bowls and serve.

Nutrition: Calories: 131, Fat: 11.2, Fiber: 1.8, Carbohydrates: 7.4, Protein: 2.1

Zucchini and Avocado Soup

Prep Time: 10 minutes **Cook Time:** 15 minutes
Servings: 4

Ingredients:
1 big avocado, pitted, peeled, and chopped
4 scallions, chopped
1 teaspoon fresh ginger, grated
2 tablespoons avocado oil
Salt and ground black pepper, to taste
2 zucchini, chopped
29 ounces vegetable stock
1 garlic clove, peeled and minced
1 cup water
1 tablespoon lemon juice
1 red bell pepper, seeded and chopped

Directions:
1.Heat a saucepan with the over medium heat, add onions, stir, and cook for 3 minutes.
2.Add garlic and ginger, stir, and cook for 1 minute.
3.Add zucchini, salt, pepper, water, stock, stir, bring to a boil, cover the pan, and cook for 10 minutes.
4.Take off heat, set soup aside for a couple of minutes, add avocado, stir, blend everything using an immersion blender, and heat up again.
5.Add more salt and pepper, plus the bell pepper and lemon juice, stir, heat up soup again, ladle into soup bowls, and serve.

Nutrition: Calories: 155, Fat: 11.1, Fiber: 6.4, Carbohydrates: 13.5, Protein: 3.7

Swiss Chard Pie

Prep Time: 10 minutes **Cook Time:** 45 minutes
Servings: 12

Ingredients:
8 cups Swiss chard, chopped
½ cup onion, peeled and chopped
1 tablespoon olive oil
1 garlic clove, peeled and minced
Salt and ground black pepper, to taste
3 eggs
2 cups ricotta cheese
1 cup mozzarella cheese, shredded
A pinch of nutmeg
¼ cup Parmesan cheese, grated
1 pound sausage, chopped

Directions:
1.Heat a pan with oil over medium heat, add onions and garlic, stir, and cook for 3 minutes.
2.Add Swiss chard, stir, and cook for 5 minutes.
3.Add salt, pepper, nutmeg, stir, take off heat, and set aside for a few minutes.
4.In a bowl, whisk eggs with cheeses and stir well.
5.Add Swiss chard mixture and stir well.
6.Spread sausage meat on the bottom of a pie pan and press well.
7.Add Swiss chard, eggs mixture, spread well, place in an oven at 350ºF and bake for 35 minutes.
8.Set the pie aside to cool down, slice, and serve it.

Nutrition: Calories: 232, Fat: 27.3, Fiber: 0.5, Carbohydrates: 3.8, Protein:15.4

Swiss Chard Salad

Prep Time: 10 minutes **Cook Time:** 20 minutes
Servings: 4

Ingredients:
1 bunch Swiss chard, cut into strips
2 tablespoons avocado oil
1 onion, peeled and chopped
A pinch of red pepper flakes
¼ cup pine nuts, toasted
1 tablespoon balsamic vinegar
Salt and ground black pepper, to taste

Directions:
1.Heat a pan with oil over medium heat, add chard and onions, stir, and cook for 5 minutes.
2.Add salt, pepper, and pepper flakes, stir, and cook for 3 minutes.
3.Add pine nuts to the pan with vinegar, stir, cook for 3 minutes, divide on plates, and serve.

Nutrition: Calories: 80, Fat: 6.8, Fiber: 1.4, Carbohydrates: 4.6, Protein: 1.8

Green Salad

Prep Time: 10 minutes **Cook Time:** 0 minutes
Servings: 4

Ingredients:
1 bunch Swiss chard, chopped
1 avocado, pitted, peeled, and cubed
Salt and ground black pepper, to taste
2 tablespoons avocado oil
1 tablespoon mustard
7 sage leaves, chopped
1 garlic clove, peeled and minced

Directions:
1.In a salad bowl, mix Swiss chard with avocado cubes. In a bowl, mix mustard with oil, sage, garlic, salt, pepper, and whisk.
2.Add this to salad, toss to coat, and serve.

Nutrition: Calories: 125, Fat: 11.3, Fiber: 4, Carbohydrates: 6, Protein: 1.9

Catalan–style Greens

Prep Time: 10 minutes **Cook Time:** 15 minutes
Servings: 4

Ingredients:
1 onion, peeled and sliced
3 tablespoons avocado oil
¼ cup prunes
6 garlic cloves, peeled and chopped
¼ cup pine nuts, toasted
¼ cup balsamic vinegar
2½ cups Swiss chard
2½ cups spinach
Salt and ground black pepper, to taste
A pinch of nutmeg

Directions:
1.Heat a pan with oil over medium–high heat, add onion, stir, and cook for 7 minutes.
2.Add garlic, stir, and cook for 1 minute.
3.Add chopped prunes, vinegar, spinach, chard, stir, and cook for 5 minutes.
4.Add nutmeg, salt, pepper, stir, cook for a few seconds, divide on plates, and serve.

Nutrition: Calories: 154, Fat: 7.8, Fiber: 5.5, Carbohydrates: 19.1, Protein: 6.1

Swiss Chard and Vegetable Soup

Prep Time: 10 minutes **Cook Time:** 2 hours and 10 minutes
Servings: 7

Ingredients:
1 onion, peeled and chopped
1 bunch Swiss chard, chopped
1 summer squash, chopped
1 zucchini, chopped
1 green bell pepper, seeded and chopped
Salt and ground black pepper, to taste
8 oz butternut squash, peeled and chopped
4 cups tomatoes, cored and chopped
1 cup cauliflower florets, chopped
1 cup green beans, chopped
6 cups chicken stock
7 ounces canned tomato paste
2 cups water
1 pound sausage, chopped
2 garlic cloves, peeled and minced
2 teaspoons thyme, chopped
1 teaspoon dried rosemary
1 tablespoon fennel, minced
½ teaspoon red pepper flakes
Some grated Parmesan cheese, for serving

Directions:
1.Heat a pan over medium–high heat, add sausage and garlic, stir and cook until it browns, and transfer along with its juices to a slow cooker.
2.Add onion, Swiss chard, summer squash, bell pepper, zucchini, butternut squash, tomatoes, cauliflower, green beans, tomato paste, stock, water, thyme, fennel, rosemary, pepper flakes, salt, pepper, stir, cover, and cook on high for 2 hours.
3.Uncover slow cooker, stir soup, ladle into bowls, sprinkle Parmesan cheese on top, and serve.

Nutrition: Calories: 324, Fat: 19.6, Fiber: 5.7, Carbohydrates: 22.4, Protein: 17.7

Swiss Chard and Chicken Soup

Prep Time: 10 minutes **Cook Time:** 35 minutes
Servings: 12

Ingredients:
4 cups Swiss chard, chopped
4 cups chicken breast, cooked, and shredded
2 cups water
1 cup mushrooms, sliced
1 tablespoon garlic, minced
1 tablespoon coconut oil, melted
¼ cup onion, peeled and chopped
8 cups chicken stock
2 cups butternut squash, chopped
1 cup green beans, cut into medium–sized pieces
2 tablespoons vinegar
¼ cup fresh basil, chopped
Salt and ground black pepper, to taste
4 bacon slices, chopped
¼ cup sundried tomatoes, cored and chopped

Directions:
1.Heat a saucepan with oil over medium–high heat, add bacon, stir, and cook for 2 minutes.
2.Add tomatoes, garlic, onions, mushrooms, stir, and cook for 5 minutes.
3.Add water, stock, chicken, stir, and cook for 15 minutes.
4.Add Swiss chard, green beans, butternut squash, salt, pepper, stir, and cook for 10 minutes.
5.Add vinegar, basil, salt, pepper, stir, ladle into soup bowls, and serve.

Nutrition: Calories: 126, Fat: 5.4, Fiber: 1.3, Carbohydrates: 5.7, Protein: 13.7

Roasted Tomato Cream

Prep Time: 10 minutes **Cook Time:** 1 hour
Servings: 8

Ingredients:
1 jalapeño pepper, chopped
4 garlic cloves, peeled and minced
2 pounds cherry tomatoes, cut in half
1 onion, peeled and cut into wedges
Salt and ground black pepper, to taste
¼ cup olive oil
½ teaspoon dried oregano
4 cups chicken stock
¼ cup fresh basil, chopped
½ cup Parmesan cheese, grated

Directions:
1.Spread tomatoes and onion in a baking dish.
2.Add garlic and chili pepper, season with salt, pepper, oregano, and drizzle oil.
3.Toss to coat and bake in oven at 425ºF for 30 minutes.
4.Take tomato mixture out of oven, transfer to a saucepan, add stock, and heat everything over medium–high heat.
5.Bring to a boil, cover the pan, reduce heat, and simmer for 20 minutes.
6.Blend using an immersion blender, add salt and pepper to taste and basil.
7.Stir, and ladle into soup bowls. Sprinkle with Parmesan cheese on top and serve.

Nutrition: Calories: 133, Fat: 9.9, Fiber: 1.8, Carbohydrates: 7.2, Protein: 6.1

Eggplant Soup

Prep Time: 10 minutes **Cook Time:** 50 minutes
Servings: 4

Ingredients:
4 tomatoes
1 teaspoon garlic, minced
¼ onion, peeled and chopped
Salt and ground black pepper, to taste
2 cups chicken stock
1 bay leaf
½ cup heavy cream
2 tablespoons fresh basil, chopped
4 tablespoons Parmesan cheese, grated
1 tablespoon olive oil
1 eggplant, chopped

Directions:
1.Spread eggplant pieces on a baking sheet, mix with oil, onion, garlic, salt, pepper, place in oven at 400ºF and bake for 15 minutes.
2.Put water in a saucepan, bring to a boil over medium heat, add tomatoes, steam for 1 minute, peel and chop.
3.Take eggplant mixture out of the oven, and transfer to a saucepan.
4.Add tomatoes, stock, bay leaf, salt, pepper, stir, bring to a boil, and simmer for 30 minutes.
5.Add heavy cream, basil, Parmesan cheese, stir, ladle into soup bowls, and serve.

Nutrition: Calories: 164, Fat: 11.3, Fiber: 5.7, Carbohydrates: 13.5, Protein: 5.3

Eggplant Stew

Prep Time: 10 minutes **Cook Time:** 30 minutes
Servings: 4

Ingredients:
1 onion, peeled and chopped
2 garlic cloves, peeled and chopped
1 bunch fresh parsley, chopped
Salt and ground black pepper, to taste
1 teaspoon dried oregano
2 eggplants, cut into medium–sized chunks
2 tablespoons olive oil
2 tablespoons capers, chopped
12 green olives, pitted and sliced
5 tomatoes, cored and chopped
3 tablespoons herb vinegar

Directions:
1.Heat a saucepan with oil over medium heat, add eggplant, oregano, salt, pepper, stir, and cook for 5 minutes.
2.Add garlic, onion, parsley, stir, and cook for 4 minutes.
3.Add capers, olives, vinegar, tomatoes, stir, and cook for 15 minutes.
4.Add more salt and pepper if needed, stir, divide into bowls, and serve.

Nutrition: Calories: 280, Fat: 17.9, Fiber: 14, Carbohydrates: 28.9, Protein: 5.4

Roasted Bell Peppers Soup

Prep Time: 10 minutes **Cook Time:** 15 minutes
Servings: 6

Ingredients:
12 ounces roasted bell peppers, seeded and chopped
2 tablespoons olive oil
2 garlic cloves, peeled and minced
29 ounces canned chicken stock
Salt and ground black pepper, to taste
7 ounces water
⅔ cup heavy cream
1 onion, peeled and chopped
¼ cup Parmesan cheese, grated
2 celery stalks, chopped

Directions:
1.Heat a saucepan with oil over medium heat, add onion, garlic, celery, some salt and pepper, stir, and cook for 8 minutes.
2.Add bell peppers, water, stock, stir, bring to a boil, cover, reduce heat and simmer for 5 minutes.
3.Use an immersion blender to puree the soup, then add more salt, pepper, cream, stir, bring to a boil and take off the heat.
4.Ladle into bowls, sprinkle Parmesan cheese, and serve.

Nutrition: Calories: 15, Fat: 12, Fiber: 2, Carbohydrates: 8.6, Protein: 4.7

Cabbage Soup

Prep Time: 10 minutes **Cook Time:** 45 minutes
Servings: 8

Ingredients:
1 garlic clove, peeled and minced
1 cabbage head, chopped
2 pounds ground beef
1 onion, peeled and chopped
1 teaspoon cumin
4 bouillon cubes
Salt and ground black pepper, to taste
10 ounces canned tomatoes, and green chilies
4 cups water

Directions:
1.Heat a pan over medium heat, add beef, stir, and brown for a few minutes.
2.Add onion, stir, cook for 4 minutes, transfer to a saucepan.
3.Heat saucepan, add cabbage, cumin, garlic, bouillon cubes, tomatoes, chilies, water, stir, bring to a boil over high heat, cover, reduce temperature and cook for 40 minutes.
4.Season with salt and pepper, stir, ladle into soup bowls, and serve.

Nutrition: Calories: 251, Fat: 7.5, Fiber: 3, Carbohydrates: 8.5, Protein: 36.4

Dessert

Coconut Pudding

Prep Time: 10 minutes **Cook Time:** 10 minutes **Servings:** 4

Ingredients:
1 and ⅔ cups coconut milk
1 tablespoon gelatin
6 tablespoons swerve
3 egg yolks
½ teaspoon vanilla extract

Directions:
1.In a bowl, mix gelatin with 1 tablespoon coconut milk, stir well, and set aside.
2.Put rest of the milk into a pan and heat over medium heat.
3.Add swerve, stir, and cook for 5 minutes.
4.In a bowl, mix egg yolks with hot coconut milk, and vanilla extract, stir well, and return everything to pan.
5.Cook for 4 minutes, add gelatin, and stir well.
6.Divide into 4 ramekins, and keep the pudding in the refrigerator until you serve it.

Nutrition: Calories: 278, Fat: 27.2, Fiber: 2.2, Carbohydrates: 13.6, Protein: 5.8

Creamy Coconut Pudding

Prep Time: 4 hours and 10 minutes **Cook Time:** 3 minutes **Servings:** 2

Ingredients:
4 teaspoons gelatin
¼ teaspoon liquid stevia
1 cup coconut milk
A pinch of ground cardamom
¼ teaspoon ground ginger
A pinch of ground nutmeg

Directions:
1.In a bowl, mix ¼ cup milk with gelatin, and stir well.
2.Put rest of the coconut milk in a saucepan and heat over medium heat.
3.Add gelatin mixture, stir, take off heat, set aside to cool down, and then keep in the refrigerator for 4 hours.
4.Transfer to a food processor, add stevia, cardamom, nutmeg, ginger, and blend for a couple of minutes.
5.Divide into dessert cups and serve cold.

Nutrition: Calories: 323, Fat: 28.6, Fiber: 2.6, Carbohydrates: 6.7, Protein: 14.7

Chocolate Biscotti

Prep Time: 10 minutes **Cook Time:** 12 minutes **Servings:** 8

Ingredients:
2 tablespoons chia seeds
2 cups almonds
1 egg
¼ cup coconut oil
¼ cup coconut, shredded
2 tablespoons stevia
¼ cup cocoa powder
A pinch of salt
1 teaspoon baking soda

Directions:
1.In a food processor, mix chia seeds with almonds and blend well.
2.Add coconut, egg, coconut oil, cocoa powder, a pinch of salt, baking soda, and stevia, and blend well.
3.Shape 8 biscotti pieces out of dough, place on a lined baking sheet, place in an oven at 350ºF and bake for 12 minutes.
4.Serve warm or cold.

Nutrition: Calories: 236, Fat: 21.5, Fiber: 5.2, Carbohydrates: 8.5, Protein: 6.9

Peanut Butter and Chocolate Brownies

Prep Time: 10 minutes **Cook Time:** 30 minutes
Servings: 4

Ingredients:
1 egg
⅓ cup cocoa powder
⅓ cup erythritol
7 tablespoons butter
A pinch of salt
½ teaspoon vanilla extract
¼ cup almond flour
¼ cup walnuts
½ teaspoon baking powder
1 tablespoon peanut butter

Directions:
1.Heat a pan with 6 tablespoons butter and erythritol over medium heat, stir, and cook for 5 minutes.
2.Transfer to a bowl, add salt, vanilla extract, cocoa powder, and whisk.
3.Add egg and stir well. Add baking powder, walnuts, almond flour, stir well, and pour into a skillet.
4.In a bowl, mix 1 tablespoon butter with peanut butter, heat in a microwave for a few seconds, and stir well.
5.Drizzle over brownie mixture in the skillet, place in an oven at 350ºF, and bake for 30 minutes.
6.Let the brownies cool down, cut, and serve.

Nutrition: Calories: 300, Fat: 30.2, Fiber: 3.2, Carbohydrates: 9.1, Protein: 6.4

Blueberry Scones

Prep Time: 10 minutes **Cook Time:** 10 minutes
Servings: 10

Ingredients:
½ cup coconut flour
1 cup blueberries
2 eggs
½ cup heavy cream
½ cup butter
½ cup almond flour
A pinch of salt
5 tablespoons stevia
2 teaspoons vanilla extract
2 teaspoons baking powder

Directions:
1.In a bowl, mix almond flour with coconut flour, salt, baking powder, blueberries, and stir well.
2.In another bowl, mix heavy cream with butter, vanilla extract, stevia, eggs, and stir well.
3.Combine the 2 mixtures, and stir until you obtain a dough.
4.Shape 10 triangles from mixture, place on a lined baking sheet, place in an oven at 350ºF and bake for 10 minutes. Serve cold.

Nutrition: Calories: 199, Fat: 16.1, Fiber: 5.2, Carbohydrates: 10.6, Protein: 4

Chocolate Cookies

Prep Time: 10 minutes **Cook Time:** 40 minutes
Servings: 12

Ingredients:
1 teaspoon vanilla extract
½ cup butter
1 egg
2 tablespoons monk fruit sweetener
¼ cup swerve
A pinch of salt
2 cups almond flour
½ cup unsweetened chocolate chips

Directions:
1.Heat a pan with butter over medium heat, stir, and cook until it browns. Take off heat and set aside for 5 minutes.
2.In a bowl, mix egg with vanilla extract, monk fruit extract, swerve, and stir.
3.Add melted butter, flour, salt, half of the chocolate chips, and stir.
4.Transfer to a pan, spread rest of the chocolate chips on top, place in an oven at 350ºF and bake for 30 minutes.
5.Slice when cool and serve.

Nutrition: Calories: 172, Fat: 15.8, Fiber: 1.8, Carbohydrates: 3.8, Protein: 3.4

Walnut Spread

Prep Time: 10 minutes **Cook Time:** 0 minutes
Servings: 6

Ingredients:
2 ounces coconut oil
4 tablespoons cocoa powder
1 teaspoon vanilla extract
1 cup walnuts, halved
4 tablespoons stevia

Directions:
1.In a food processor, mix cocoa powder with oil, vanilla extract, walnuts, stevia, and blend well.
2.Keep in refrigerator for a couple of hours and serve.

Nutrition: Calories: 220, Fat: 22.2, Fiber: 2.5, Carbohydrates: 4.1, Protein: 5.7

Mug Cake

Prep Time: 2 minutes **Cook Time:** 3 minutes
Servings: 1

Ingredients:
4 tablespoons almond meal
2 tablespoon butter
1 teaspoon stevia
1 tablespoon cocoa powder, unsweetened
1 egg
1 tablespoon coconut flour
¼ teaspoon vanilla extract
½ teaspoon baking powder

Directions:
1.Put the butter in a mug and place in microwave for a couple of seconds.
2.Add cocoa powder, stevia, egg, baking powder, vanilla extract, coconut flour, and stir well.
3.Add almond meal, stir again, place back in the microwave, cook for 2 minutes.
4.Serve the mug cake with berries on top.

Nutrition: Calories: 476, Fat: 41.5, Fiber: 10.6, Carbohydrates: 18.4, Protein: 13.8

Sweet Buns

Prep Time: 10 minutes **Cook Time:** 30 minutes
Servings: 8

Ingredients:
½ cup coconut flour
⅓ cup psyllium husks
2 tablespoons swerve
1 teaspoon baking powder
A pinch of salt
½ teaspoon ground cinnamon
½ teaspoon ground cloves
4 eggs
Chocolate chips, unsweetened
1 cup hot water

Directions:
1.In a bowl, mix flour with psyllium husks, swerve, baking powder, salt, cinnamon, cloves, chocolate chips, and stir well.
2.Add water and egg, stir well until you obtain a dough, shape 8 buns, and arrange on a lined baking sheet.
3.Place in oven at 350ºF and bake for 30 minutes. Let cool and serve.

Nutrition: Calories: 141, Fat: 3.5, Fiber: 24.1, Carbohydrates: 31.6, Protein: 4.5

Chocolate Ganache

Prep Time: 1 minute **Cook Time:** 5 minutes
Servings: 6

Ingredients:
½ cup heavy cream
4 ounces dark chocolate, unsweetened, and chopped

Directions:
1.Put the cream in a pan and heat over medium heat.
2.Take off heat when it begins to simmer, add the chocolate pieces, and stir until it melts.
3.Serve cold as a dessert or use it as a topping for a keto cake.

Nutrition: Calories: 136, Fat: 9.3, Fiber: 0.6, Carbohydrates: 11.5, Protein: 1.7

Lemon Custard

Prep Time: 10 minutes **Cook Time:** 30 minutes
Servings: 6

Ingredients:
1⅓pint almond milk
4 tablespoons lemon zest
4 eggs
5 tablespoons swerve
2 tablespoons lemon juice

Directions:
1.In a bowl, mix eggs with milk and swerve and stir well.
2.Add lemon zest and lemon juice, whisk, pour into ramekins, and place into a baking dish with some water on the bottom.
3.Bake in the oven at 360ºF for 30 minutes.
4.Let the custard cool before serving.

Nutrition: Calories: 111, Fat: 5.7, Fiber: 0.3, Carbohydrates: 14, Protein: 4.9

Peach Cake

Prep Time: 10 minutes **Cook Time:** 20 minutes
Servings: 12

Ingredients:
6 eggs
2 peaches, stoned, cut into quarters
1 teaspoon vanilla extract
1 teaspoon baking powder
9 ounces almond meal
4 tablespoons swerve
A pinch of salt
2 tablespoons orange zest
2 ounces stevia
4 ounces cream cheese
4 ounces coconut yogurt

Directions:
In a food processor, pulse peaches well.
Add almond meal, swerve, eggs, baking powder, vanilla extract, a pinch of salt, and pulse well.
1.Transfer into 2 springform pans, place in an oven at 350ºF and bake for 20 minutes.
2.In a bowl, mix cream cheese with orange zest, coconut yogurt, stevia, and stir well.
3.Place one cake layer on a plate, add half of the cream cheese mixture, add the other cake layer, and top with the rest of the cream cheese mixture.
4.Spread it well, slice, and serve.

Nutrition: Calories: 207, Fat: 16.5, Fiber: 3.1, Carbohydrates: 8.6, Protein: 8.7

Mixed Berries and Cream

Prep Time: 10 minutes **Cook Time:** 0 minutes
Servings: 4

Ingredients:
3 tablespoons cocoa powder
14 ounces heavy cream
1 cup blackberries
1 cup raspberries
2 tablespoons stevia
Coconut chips

Directions:
1.In a bowl, whisk cocoa powder with stevia and heavy cream.
2.Divide some mixture into dessert bowls, add blackberries, raspberries, and coconut chips, then spread another layer of cream, and top with berries and chips. Serve cold.

Nutrition: Calories: 383, Fat: 37.6, Fiber: 5.1, Carbohydrates: 12.1, Protein: 3.6

Coconut Ice Cream

Prep Time: 10 minutes **Cook Time:** 0 minutes
Servings: 8

Ingredients:
1 papaya, sliced
14 ounces coconut cream, frozen

Directions:
1.In a food processor, mix papaya with cream and pulse well.
2.Divide into bowls and serve.

Nutrition: Calories:131, Fat: 13.5, Fiber: 1.8, Carbohydrates: 7, Protein: 1.3

Macaroons

Prep Time: 10 minutes **Cook Time:** 10 minutes
Servings: 20

Ingredients:
2 tablespoons stevia
4 egg whites
2 cup coconut, shredded
1 teaspoon vanilla extract

Directions:
1.In a bowl, mix egg whites with stevia and beat using a mixer.
2.Add coconut and vanilla extract and stir.
3.Roll mixture into small balls and place them on a lined baking sheet.
4.Place in oven at 350ºF and bake for 10 minutes. Cool and serve.

Nutrition: Calories: 32, Fat: 2.7, Fiber: 0.7, Carbohydrates: 1.3, Protein: 1

Lime Cheesecake

Prep Time: 10 minutes **Cook Time:** 2 minutes
Servings: 10

Ingredients:
2 tablespoons butter, melted
2 teaspoons granulated stevia
4 ounces almond meal
¼ cup coconut, unsweetened, and shredded
For the filling:
1 pound cream cheese
Zest from 1 lime
Juice from 1 lime
2 sachets sugar–free lime jelly
2 cup hot water

Directions:
1.Heat a small pan over medium heat, add butter, and stir until it melts.
2.In a bowl, mix coconut with almond meal, butter, stevia, and stir well.
3.Press this on bottom of a round pan, and place in refrigerator.
4.Put hot water in a bowl, add jelly sachets, and stir until it dissolves.
5.Put cream cheese in a bowl, add jelly, and stir well.
6.Add lime juice, lime zest and blend using a mixer.
7.Pour over the base, spread, and keep the cheesecake in the refrigerator until you serve it.

Nutrition: Calories: 253, Fat: 24.5, Fiber: 1.8, Carbohydrates: 4.7, Protein: 6

Caramel Custard

Prep Time: 10 minutes **Cook Time:** 30 minutes
Servings: 2

Ingredients:
1½ teaspoons caramel extract
1 cup water
2 ounces cream cheese
2 eggs
1½ tablespoons swerve
For the caramel sauce:
2 tablespoons swerve
2 tablespoons butter
¼ teaspoon caramel extract

Directions:
1.In a blender, mix cream cheese with water, 1½ tablespoons swerve, 1½ teaspoons caramel extract, eggs, and blend well.
2.Pour into 2 greased ramekins, place in oven at 350ºF and bake for 30 minutes.
3.Put butter in a saucepan and heat over medium heat.
4.Add ¼ teaspoon caramel extract and 2 tablespoons swerve, stir well, and cook until everything melts.
5.Pour over caramel custard, let cool, and serve.

Nutrition: Calories: 372, Fat: 31, Fiber: 0.1, Carbohydrates: 11.3, Protein: 8.9

Coconut and Strawberries

Prep Time: 10 minutes **Cook Time:** 0 minutes
Servings: 4

Ingredients:
1¾ cups coconut cream
2 teaspoons granulated stevia
1 cup strawberries

Directions:
1.Put coconut cream in a bowl, add stevia, and stir well using an immersion blender.
2.Add strawberries, fold them gently into mixture, divide dessert into glasses, and serve them cold.

Nutrition: Calories: 460, Fat: 46.6, Fiber: 5, Carbohydrates: 13.6, Protein: 4.7

Chocolate Truffles

Prep Time: 10 minutes **Cook Time:** 6 minutes
Servings: 22

Ingredients:
1 cup sugar–free chocolate chips
2 tablespoons butter
⅔ cup heavy cream
2 teaspoons brandy
2 tablespoons swerve
¼ teaspoon vanilla extract
Cocoa powder

Directions:
1.Put the heavy cream in a heatproof bowl, add swerve, butter, chocolate chips, stir, place in a microwave and heat for 1 minute.
2.Set aside for 5 minutes, stir well, and mix with brandy and vanilla extract.
3.Stir again and set aside in refrigerator for a couple of hours.
4.Use a melon baller to shape the truffles, roll them in cocoa powder, and serve.

Nutrition: Calories: 62, Fat: 4.4, Fiber: 0, Carbohydrates: 6.3, Protein: 0.5

Berry Mousse

Prep Time: 10 minutes **Cook Time:** 0 minutes
Servings: 12

Ingredients:
8 ounces mascarpone cheese
¾ teaspoon stevia
½ teaspoon vanilla extract
1 cup whipping cream
½ pint blueberries
½ pint strawberries

Directions:
1.In a bowl, mix whipping cream with stevia, mascarpone, and blend well using a mixer.
2.Arrange a layer of blueberries and strawberries in 12 glasses, then a layer of cream, and repeat. Serve cold.

Nutrition: Calories: 77, Fat: 5.6, Fiber: 0.7, Carbohydrates: 2.8, Protein: 4.6

Chocolate Bombs

Prep Time: 10 minutes **Cook Time:** 10 minutes
Servings: 12

Ingredients:
10 tablespoons coconut oil
3 tablespoons macadamia nuts, chopped
2 packets stevia
5 tablespoons unsweetened coconut powder
A pinch of salt

Directions:
1.Put coconut oil in a saucepan and melt over medium heat.
2.Add stevia, salt, cocoa powder, stir well, and take off heat.
3.Spoon into a candy tray and keep in refrigerator for a couple of hours.
4.Sprinkle macadamia nuts on top and keep in the refrigerator until ready to serve.

Nutrition: Calories: 137, Fat: 15.2, Fiber: 0.2, Carbohydrates: 1.1, Protein: 0.4

Creamy Jelly

Prep Time: 2 hours 10 minutes **Cook Time:** 5 minutes
Servings: 12

Ingredients:
2 ounces packets sugar–free gelatin
1 cup cold water
1 cup hot water
3 tablespoons erythritol
2 tablespoons gelatin powder
1 teaspoon vanilla extract
1 cup heavy cream
1 cup boiling water

Directions:
1.Open gelatin packets, put gelatin powder in a bowl, add 1 cup hot water, stir until dissolved, and then mix with 1 cup cold water.
2.Pour into a lined square dish and keep in refrigerator for 1 hour. Cut into cubes and set aside.
3.In a bowl, mix erythritol with vanilla extract, 1 cup boiling water, gelatin, heavy cream, and stir well.
4.Pour half of this mix into a silicon round mold, spread gelatin cubes, and then top with rest of the gelatin.
5.Keep in the refrigerator for 1 more hour and then serve.

Nutrition: Calories: 39, Fat: 3.7, Fiber: 0, Carbohydrates: 7.31, Protein: 1.2

Doughnuts

Prep Time: 10 minutes **Cook Time:** 15 minutes
Servings: 24

Ingredients:
¼ cup erythritol
¼ cup flaxseed meal
¾ cup almond flour
1 teaspoon baking powder
1 teaspoon vanilla extract
2 eggs
3 tablespoons coconut oil
¼ cup coconut milk
20 drops red food coloring
A pinch of salt
1 tablespoon cocoa powder

Directions:
1.In a bowl, mix flaxseed meal with almond flour, cocoa powder, baking powder, erythritol, salt, and stir.
2.In another bowl, mix coconut oil with coconut milk, vanilla extract, food coloring, eggs, and stir.
3.Combine 2 mixtures, stir using a hand mixer, transfer to a piping bag, make a hole in the bag, and shape 12 doughnuts on a baking sheet.
4.Place in an oven at 350ºF and bake for 15 minutes. Arrange them on a platter and serve.

Nutrition: Calories: 41, Fat: 3.7, Fiber: 0.5, Carbohydrates: 3, Protein: 1

Chocolate Cups

Prep Time: 30 minutes **Cook Time:** 5 minutes
Servings: 20

Ingredients:
½ cup coconut butter
½ cup coconut oil
3 tablespoons swerve
½ cup coconut, shredded
1. 5 ounces cocoa butter
1 ounces chocolate, unsweetened
¼ cup cocoa powder
¼ teaspoon vanilla extract
¼ cup swerve

Directions:
1.In a pan, mix coconut butter with coconut oil, stir, and heat up over medium heat.
2.Add coconut and 3 tablespoons swerve, stir well, take off heat, scoop into a lined muffins pan, and keep in refrigerator for 30 minutes.
3.In a bowl, mix cocoa butter with chocolate, vanilla extract, ¼ cup swerve, and stir well.
4.Place this over a bowl filled with boiling water and stir until everything is smooth.
5.Spoon over coconut cupcakes, keep in the refrigerator for 15 minutes, and then serve.

Nutrition: Calories: 201, Fat: 21.2, Fiber: 1.8, Carbohydrates: 4.2, Protein: 0.9

Brownies

Prep Time: 10 minutes **Cook Time:** 20 minutes **Servings:** 12

Ingredients:
6 ounces coconut oil, melted
6 eggs
3 ounces cocoa powder
2 teaspoons vanilla extract
½ teaspoon baking powder
4 ounces cream cheese
5 tablespoons swerve

Directions:
1.In a blender, mix eggs with coconut oil, cocoa powder, baking powder, vanilla extract, cream cheese, swerve and stir using a mixer.
2.Pour into a lined baking dish, place in an oven at 350ºF and bake for 20 minutes.
3.Cool then slice into rectangle pieces, and serve.

Nutrition: Calories: 202, Fat: 20.6, Fiber: 2.1, Carbohydrates: 4.3, Protein: 4.8

Chocolate Pie

Prep Time: 3 hours 10 minutes **Cook Time:** 20 minutes **Servings:** 10

Ingredients:
For the crust:
½ teaspoon baking powder
1½ cup almond crust
A pinch of salt
⅓ cup stevia
1 egg
1½ teaspoons vanilla extract
3 tablespoons butter
1 teaspoon butter for the pan
For the filling:
1 tablespoon vanilla extract
4 tablespoons butter
4 tablespoons sour cream
16 ounces cream cheese
½ cup cut stevia
½ cup cocoa powder
2 teaspoons granulated stevia
1 cup whipping cream
1 teaspoon vanilla extract

Directions:
1.Grease a springform pan with 1 teaspoon butter and set aside.
2.In a bowl, mix baking powder with ⅓ cup stevia, a pinch of salt and almond flour, and stir.
3.Add 3 tablespoons butter, egg, and 1½ teaspoon vanilla extract, stir until you obtain a dough.
4.Press well into springform pan, place in oven at 375ºF, and bake for 11 minutes.
5.Take pie crust out of oven, cover with aluminum foil and bake for 8 minutes.
6.Take it out of oven and set aside to cool down.
7.In a bowl, mix cream cheese with 4 tablespoons butter, sour cream, 1 tablespoon vanilla extract, cocoa powder, ½ cup stevia, and stir well.
8.In another bowl, mix whipping cream with 2 teaspoons stevia, 1 teaspoon vanilla extract, and stir using a mixer.
9.Combine 2 mixtures, pour into pie crust, spread well, place in refrigerator for 3 hours and then serve.

Nutrition: Calories: 313, Fat: 29.9, Fiber: 2.3, Carbohydrates: 6.7, Protein:7.2

Lemon Mousse

Prep Time: 10 minutes **Cook Time:** 0 minutes **Servings:** 5

Ingredients:
1 cup heavy cream
A pinch of salt
1 teaspoon stevia
½ cup lemon juice
8 ounces mascarpone cheese

Directions:
1.In a bowl, mix heavy cream with mascarpone and lemon juice, and stir using a mixer.
2.Add a pinch of salt, stevia, and blend everything.
3.Divide into dessert glasses and keep in the refrigerator until ready to serve.

Nutrition: Calories: 168, Fat: 15, Fiber: 0.1, Carbohydrates: 2.6, Protein: 5.8

Strawberry Pie

Prep Time: 2 hours and 10 minutes **Cook Time:** 5 minutes
Servings: 12

Ingredients:
For the crust:
1 cup coconut, shredded
1 cup sunflower seeds
¼ cup butter
A pinch of salt
For the filling:
1 teaspoon gelatin
8 ounces cream cheese
4 ounces strawberries
2 tablespoons water
½ tablespoon lemon juice
¼ teaspoon stevia
½ cup heavy cream
8 ounces strawberries, hulled, and chopped, for serving
16 ounces heavy cream, for serving

Directions:
1.In a food processor, mix sunflower seeds with coconut, a pinch of salt, butter, and stir well.
2.Put into a greased springform pan and press well on the bottom.
3.Heat a pan with water over medium heat, add gelatin, stir until it dissolves, take off heat, and set aside to cool down.
4.Add to a food processor, mix with 4 ounces strawberries, cream cheese, lemon juice, stevia, and blend well.
5.Add ½ cup heavy cream, stir well, spread over crust.
6.Top with 8 ounces strawberries, 16 ounces heavy cream and keep in the refrigerator for 2 hours before slicing and serving.

Nutrition: Calories: 201, Fat: 20.2, Fiber: 1.1, Carbohydrates: 3.4, Protein: 2.9

Summer Smoothie

Prep Time: 5 minutes **Cook Time:** 0 minutes
Servings: 4

Ingredients:
½ cup coconut milk
1½ cup avocado, pitted and peeled
2 tablespoons green tea powder
2 teaspoons lime zest
1 tablespoon stevia

Directions:
1.In a smoothie maker, combine milk with avocado, green tea powder, lime zest, and pulse well.
2.Add stevia, blend well, divide into 2 glasses, and serve.

Nutrition: Calories: 481, Fat: 46.3, Fiber: 14.7, Carbohydrates: 19.1, Protein: 5

Vanilla Ice Cream

Prep Time: 3 hours and 10 minutes **Cook Time:** 0 minutes
Servings: 6

Ingredients:
4 eggs, yolks, and whites separated
¼ teaspoon cream of tartar
½ cup swerve
1 tablespoon vanilla extract
1¼ cup heavy whipping cream

Directions:
1.In a bowl, mix egg whites with cream of tartar and swerve, and stir using a mixer.
2.In another bowl, whisk cream with vanilla extract and blend well.
3.Combine 2 mixtures and stir gently.
4.In another bowl, whisk egg yolks and then add two egg whites mixture.
5.Stir gently, pour the mixture into a container, and keep in the freezer for 3 hours before serving.

Nutrition: Calories: 238, Fat: 23.3, Fiber: 0, Carbohydrates: 8.8, Protein: 4.8

Mini Cheesecakes

Prep Time: 10 minutes **Cook Time:** 15 minutes **Servings:** 9

Ingredients:
For the cheesecakes:
2 tablespoons butter
8 ounces cream cheese
3 tablespoons coffee
3 eggs
⅓ cup swerve
1 tablespoon sugar–free caramel syrup
For the frosting:
3 tablespoons sugar–free caramel syrup
3 tablespoons butter
8 ounces mascarpone cheese, softened
2 tablespoons swerve

Directions:
1.In a blender, mix cream cheese with eggs, 2 tablespoons butter, coffee, 1 tablespoon caramel syrup, ⅓ cup swerve, and pulse well.
2.Spoon into a cupcake pan, place in oven at 350ºF and bake for 15 minutes.
3.Set aside to cool down, and then keep in the freezer for 3 hours.
4.In a bowl, mix 3 tablespoons butter with 3 tablespoons caramel syrup, 2 tablespoons swerve, mascarpone cheese, and blend well.
5.Spoon this over cheesecakes and serve.

Nutrition: Calories: 166, Fat: 16.7, Fiber: 0, Carbohydrates: 37.1, Protein: 3.8

Raspberry and Coconut Dessert

Prep Time: 10 minutes **Cook Time:** 5 minutes **Servings:** 12

Ingredients:
½ cup coconut butter
½ cup coconut oil
½ cup raspberries, dried
¼ cup swerve
½ cup coconut, shredded

Directions:
1.In a food processor, blend dried berries.
2.Heat a pan with butter over medium heat. Add oil, coconut, and swerve, stir, and cook for 5 minutes.
3.Pour half into a lined baking pan and spread well.
4.Add raspberry powder and spread well.
5.Top with remaining butter mixture, spread, and keep in refrigerator for a couple of hours, then cut into pieces and serve.

Nutrition: Calories: 124, Fat: 13.1, Fiber: 1.5, Carbohydrates: 2.3, Protein: 0.5

Peanut Butter Fudge

Prep Time: 2 hours and 10 minutes **Cook Time:** 2 minutes **Servings:** 12

Ingredients:
1 cup peanut butter, unsweetened
¼ cup almond milk
½ teaspoon vanilla extract
2 teaspoons stevia
1 cup coconut oil
A pinch of salt
For the topping:
2 tablespoons swerve
2 tablespoons melted coconut oil
¼ cup cocoa powder

Directions:
1.In a heatproof bowl, mix peanut butter with 1 cup coconut oil, stir, and heat up in a microwave until it melts.
2.Add a pinch of salt, almond milk, stevia, stir well, and pour into a lined loaf pan.
3.Keep in refrigerator for 2 hours and then slice it.
4.In a bowl, mix 2 tablespoons melted coconut oil with cocoa powder, swerve, and stir well.
5.Drizzle sauce over the peanut butter fudge and serve.

Nutrition: Calories: 312, Fat: 31.9, Fiber: 1.9, Carbohydrates: 6.3, Protein: 5.8

Cheesecake Squares

Prep Time: 10 minutes **Cook Time:** 20 minutes
Servings: 9

Ingredients:
5 ounces coconut oil, melted
½ teaspoon baking powder
4 tablespoons swerve
1 teaspoon vanilla extract
4 ounces cream cheese
6 eggs
½ cup blueberries

Directions:
1.In a bowl, mix coconut oil with eggs, cream cheese, vanilla extract, swerve, baking powder and blend using an immersion blender.
2.Fold blueberries, pour everything into a square baking dish, place in an oven at 320ºF and bake for 20 minutes.
3.Let the cake cool down, slice into squares, and serve.

Nutrition: Calories: 228, Fat: 23.1, Fiber: 0.2, Carbohydrates: 4.2, Protein: 4.7

Chocolate Pudding

Prep Time: 50 minutes **Cook Time:** 5 minutes
Servings: 2

Ingredients:
2 tablespoons water
1 tablespoon gelatin
2 tablespoons erythritol
½ teaspoon stevia powder
2 tablespoons cocoa powder
1 cup coconut milk

Directions:
1.Heat a pan with coconut milk over medium heat, add stevia and cocoa powder, and stir well.
2.In a bowl, mix gelatin with water, stir well, and add to pan.
3.Stir well, add erythritol, whisk again, divide into ramekins, and keep in refrigerator for 45 minutes. Serve cold.

Nutrition: Calories: 300, Fat: 29.3, Fiber: 4.3, Carbohydrates: 9.6, Protein: 6.7

Vanilla Parfaits

Prep Time: 10 minutes **Cook Time:** 0 minutes
Servings: 4

Ingredients:
14 ounces canned coconut milk
1 teaspoon vanilla extract
10 drops stevia
4 ounces berries
2 tablespoons walnuts, chopped

Directions:
1.In a bowl, mix coconut milk with stevia and vanilla extract, and whisk using a mixer.
2.In another bowl, mix berries with walnuts and stir.
3.Spoon half of vanilla coconut mixture into 4 jars, add a layer of berries, and top with rest of the vanilla mixture.
4.Top with berries and walnuts mixture, place in the refrigerator to chill before serving.

Nutrition: Calories: 272, Fat: 26.1, Fiber: 3.5, Carbohydrates: 9.5, Protein: 3.4

Avocado Pudding

Prep Time: 10 minutes **Cook Time:** 0 minutes
Servings: 8

Ingredients:
2 avocados, pitted, peeled, and chopped
2 teaspoons vanilla extract
80 drops stevia
1 tablespoon lime juice
14 ounces canned coconut milk

Directions:
1.In a blender, mix avocado with coconut milk, vanilla extract, stevia, and lime juice, blend well, spoon into dessert bowls, and keep in the refrigerator until ready to serve it.

Nutrition: Calories: 221, Fat: 21.3, Fiber: 4.5, Carbohydrates: 7.8, Protein: 2.1

Mint Delight

Prep Time: 2 hours and 10 minutes **Cook Time:** 0 minutes **Servings:** 3

Ingredients:
½ cup coconut oil, melted
3 stevia drops
1 tablespoon cocoa powder
For the pudding:
1 teaspoon peppermint oil
14 ounces canned coconut milk
1 avocado, pitted, peeled, and chopped
10 drops stevia

Directions:
1.In a bowl, mix coconut oil with cocoa powder and 3 drops stevia, stir well, transfer to a lined container, and keep in the refrigerator for 1 hour.
2.Chop into small pieces and set aside.
3.In a blender, mix coconut milk with avocado, 10 drops stevia, peppermint oil, and pulse well.
4.Add chocolate chips, fold them gently, divide pudding into bowls, and keep in the refrigerator for an hour.

Nutrition: Calories: 758, Fat: 81.2, Fiber: 7.9, Carbohydrates: 14.1, Protein: 4.6

Cookie Dough Balls

Prep Time: 10 minutes **Cook Time:** 0 minutes **Servings:** 10

Ingredients:
½ cup almond butter
3 tablespoons coconut flour
3 tablespoons coconut milk
1 teaspoon ground cinnamon, powder
3 tablespoons coconut sugar
15 drops stevia
A pinch of salt
1 teaspoon vanilla extract
For the topping:
1½ teaspoon ground cinnamon
3 tablespoons granulated swerve

Directions:
1.In a bowl, mix almond butter with 1 teaspoon ground cinnamon, coconut flour, coconut milk, coconut sugar, vanilla extract, stevia, a pinch of salt, and stir well.
2.Shape balls out of mixture.
3.In another bowl, mix 1½ teaspoon cinnamon with swerve and stir well.
4.Roll balls in cinnamon mixture and keep in the refrigerator until you serve.

Nutrition: Calories: 35, Fat: 2, Fiber: 2.1, Carbohydrates: 3.9, Protein: 0.9

Ricotta Mousse

Prep Time: 2 hours and 10 minutes **Cook Time:** 0 minutes **Servings:** 10

Ingredients:
½ cup hot coffee
2 cups ricotta cheese
2, and ½ teaspoons gelatin
1½ teaspoon vanilla extract
1 teaspoon espresso powder
1 teaspoon stevia
A pinch of salt
1 cup whipping cream

Directions:
1.In a bowl, mix coffee with gelatin, stir well, and set aside until coffee is cold.
2.In a bowl, mix espresso, stevia, salt, vanilla extract, ricotta, and stir using a mixer.
3.Add coffee mixture and stir well. Add whipping cream and blend mixture again.
4.Divide into dessert bowls and serve after chilling in refrigerator for 2 hours.

Nutrition: Calories: 110, Fat: 7.6, Fiber: 0, Carbohydrates: 3.2, Protein: 5.9

Coconut Granola

Prep Time: 10 minutes **Cook Time:** 35 minutes
Servings: 4

Ingredients:
1 cup coconut, unsweetened, and shredded
1 cup almonds, and pecans, chopped
2 tablespoons stevia
½ cup pumpkin seeds
½ cup sunflower seeds
2 tablespoons coconut oil
1 teaspoon ground nutmeg
1/2 teaspoon cinnamon
1/8 teaspoon ground nutmeg
1/8 teaspoon ground allspice

Directions:
1.In a bowl, mix almonds, pecans, pumpkin seeds, sunflower seeds, coconut, nutmeg, 1/2 teaspoon cinnamon, 1/8 teaspoon ground nutmeg, 1/8 teaspoon ground allspice, and stir well.
2.Heat a pan with coconut oil over medium heat, add stevia, and stir until combined.
3.Pour over nuts and coconut mixture and stir well.
4.Spread on a lined baking sheet, place in oven at 300ºF and bake for 30 minutes.
5.Let granola cool, then cut and serve.

Nutrition: Calories: 394, Fat: 36.2, Fiber: 5.9, Carbohydrates: 12.4, Protein: 11.1

Peanut Butter and Chia Pudding

Prep Time: 10 minutes **Cook Time:** 0 minutes
Servings: 4

Ingredients:
½ cup chia seeds
2 cups almond milk, unsweetened
1½ teaspoon vanilla extract
¼ cup peanut butter, unsweetened
1 teaspoon stevia
A pinch of salt

Directions:
1.In a bowl, mix milk with chia seeds, peanut butter, vanilla extract, stevia, pinch of salt, and stir well.
2.Leave pudding aside for 5 minutes, then stir it again, divide into dessert glasses, and leave in refrigerator for 10 minutes before serving.

Nutrition: Calories: 456, Fat: 41.1, Fiber: 8.5, Carbohydrates: 6.5, Protein: 9.1

Pumpkin Custard

Prep Time: 10 minutes **Cook Time:** 5 minutes
Servings: 6

Ingredients:
1 tablespoon gelatin
¼ cup warm water
14 ounces canned coconut milk
14 ounces canned pumpkin puree
A pinch of salt
2 teaspoons vanilla extract
1 teaspoon ground cinnamon
1/2 teaspoon cinnamon
1/8 teaspoon cloves
1/4 teaspoon ginger
1/8 teaspoon nutmeg.
2 tablespoons stevia
3 tablespoons erythritol

Directions:
1.In a pot, mix pumpkin puree with coconut milk, a pinch of salt, vanilla extract, cinnamon, stevia, erythritol, and cinnamon, cloves, ginger, nutmeg, stir well, and heat for a couple of minutes.
2.In a bowl, mix gelatin, water, and stir.
3.Combine the 2 mixtures, stir well, divide custard into ramekins and set aside to cool down.
4.Keep in refrigerator until ready to serve.

Nutrition: Calories: 179, Fat: 16, Fiber: 3.4, Carbohydrates: 9, Protein: 3.2

Marshmallows

Prep Time: 10 minutes **Cook Time:** 3 minutes
Servings: 6

Ingredients:
2 tablespoons gelatin
12 scoops stevia
½ cup cold water
½ cup hot water
2 teaspoons vanilla extract
¾ cup erythritol

Directions:
1.In a bowl, mix gelatin with cold water, stir, and set aside for 5 minutes.
2.Put hot water in a pan, add erythritol, stevia, and stir well.
3.Combine with gelatin mixture, add vanilla extract, and stir well.
4.Beat using a mixer and pour into a baking pan.
5.Set aside in refrigerator until set, then cut into pieces, and serve.

Nutrition: Calories: 12, Fat: 0, Fiber: 0, Carbohydrates: 7.7, Protein: 2

Tiramisu Pudding

Prep Time: 2 hours and 10 minutes **Cook Time:** 0 minutes **Servings:** 10

Ingredients:
8 ounces cream cheese
16 ounces cottage cheese
2 tablespoons unsweetened cocoa powder
1 teaspoon instant coffee
4 tablespoons almond milk
½ cup erythritol

Directions:
1.In a food processor, mix cottage cheese with cream cheese, cocoa powder, coffee, and blend well.
2.Add erythritol and almond milk, blend again, and divide into dessert cups.
3.Keep in refrigerator until you are ready to serve.

Nutrition: Calories: 136.3, Fat: 10.3, Fiber: 0.5, Carbohydrates: 8.2, Protein: 8.2

Lemon Sorbet

Prep Time: 5 minutes **Cook Time:** 0 minutes
Servings: 4

Ingredients:
4 cups ice
Stevia, to taste
1 lemon, peeled, and chopped

Directions:
1.In a blender, mix lemon with stevia and ice, and blend until everything is combined.
2.Divide into glasses and serve cold.

Nutrition: Calories: 15, Fat: 0.2, Fiber: 1,5, Carbohydrates: 4.9, Protein: 0.6

No-bake Cookies

Prep Time: 40 minutes **Cook Time:** 2 minutes
Servings: 4

Ingredients:
1/5 cup swerve
¼ cup coconut milk
¼ cup coconut oil
2 tablespoons cocoa powder
1¾ cup coconut, shredded
½ teaspoon vanilla extract
A pinch of salt
¾ cup almond butter

Directions:
1.Heat a pan with oil over medium-high heat, add milk, cocoa powder, swerve, stir well for about 2 minutes, and take off heat.
2.Add vanilla extract, a pinch of salt, coconut, almond butter, and stir well.
3.Place spoonful of mixture on a lined baking sheet, keep in refrigerator for 30 minutes, and then serve them.

Nutrition: Calories: 325, Fat: 32.8, Fiber: 5.8, Carbohydrates: 17.2, Protein: 2.9

Butter Delight

Prep Time: 10 minutes **Cook Time:** 4 minutes
Servings: 16

Ingredients:
4 ounces coconut butter
4 ounces cocoa butter
¼ cup swerve
½ cup peanut butter
4 ounces dark chocolate, sugar free
½ teaspoon vanilla extract
⅛ teaspoon xanthan gum

Directions:
1.Put coconut butter, cocoa butter, peanut butter, and swerve in a pan, and heat over medium heat.
2.Stir until combined, and mix with the xanthan gum and vanilla extract.
3.Stir well, pour into a lined baking sheet, and spread in a pan.
4.Keep this in the refrigerator for 10 minutes.
5.Heat up a saucepan with water over medium–high heat and bring to a simmer.
6.Add a bowl on top of pan and add chocolate to bowl.
7.Stir until it melts and drizzle over butter mixture.
8.Keep in refrigerator until everything is firm, cut into 16 pieces, and serve.

Nutrition: Calories: 188, Fat: 16.9, Fiber: 2, Carbohydrates: 7.6, Protein: 3.1

Raspberry Ice Pops

Prep Time: 2 hours **Cook Time:** 10 minutes
Servings: 4

Ingredients:
1½ cups raspberries
2 cups water

Directions:
1.Put raspberries and water in a pan, bring to a boil, and simmer for 10 minutes at medium heat.
2.Pour mixture into an ice cube tray, stick ice pop sticks into each one, and freeze for 2 hours.

Nutrition: Calories: 24, Fat: 0.3, Fiber: 3, Carbohydrates: 5.5, Protein: 0.6

Cherry and Chia Jam

Prep Time: 15 minutes **Cook Time:** 12 minutes
Servings: 22

Ingredients:
3 tablespoons chia seeds
2, and ½ cups cherries, pitted
½ teaspoon vanilla extract
Peel from ½ lemon, grated
¼ cup erythritol
10 drops stevia
1 cup water

Directions:
1.Put cherries and water in a saucepan, add other ingredients stir, bring to a simmer, and cook for 12 minutes.
2.Set jam aside for 15 minutes.

Nutrition: Calories: 26, Fat: 0.8, Fiber: 1.4, Carbohydrates: 4.9, Protein: 0.8

Conclusion

Our cookbook will help you get started on your new, life–changing keto diet. It provides multiple recipes to help get begin your ketogenic journey.

We have compiled some of the most popular ketogenic recipes in the world. Simple, delicious and easy to make.

Congratulations on starting your new life as a follower of the ketogenic diet. You now have your hands on our delicious recipe collection, and can start cooking in this new, exciting and healthy way.

Most importantly, have fun and enjoy your ketogenic lifestyle!

Milton Keynes UK
Ingram Content Group UK Ltd.
UKHW051122231023
431175UK00013B/838